YOU ARE YOUR OWN GYM
THE COOKBOOK

BY MARK LAUREN

You Are Your Own Gym: The Cookbook

Body Fuel

You Are Your Own Gym

Body by You

YOU ARE YOUR OWN GYM
THE COOKBOOK

Protein

+

FAST FUEL

+

SLOW FUEL

Protein

+

FAST FUEL

Protein

+

SLOW FUEL

Protein

+

FAST FUEL

+

SLOW FUEL

YOU ARE YOUR OWN GYM
THE COOKBOOK

125 Delicious Recipes for Cooking Your Way to a Great Body

MARK LAUREN

WITH MAGGIE GREENWOOD-ROBINSON

Vermilion
LONDON

10 9 8 7 6 5 4 3 2 1

Vermilion, an imprint of Ebury Publishing,
20 Vauxhall Bridge Road,
London SW1V 2SA

Vermilion is part of the Penguin Random House group of companies whose addresses can be found at global.penguinrandomhouse.com

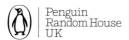
Penguin
Random House
UK

This edition published by Vermilion in arrangement with Ballantine Books, a division of Random House Inc. in 2017

www.penguin.co.uk

A CIP catalogue record for this book is available from the British Library

ISBN 9780091955403

Printed and bound in China by Leo Paper Products Ltd

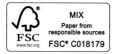

MIX
Paper from
responsible sources
FSC® C018179

Penguin Random House is committed to a sustainable future for our business, our readers and our planet. This book is made from Forest Stewardship Council® certified paper.

CONTENTS

INTRODUCTION: YOU ARE YOUR OWN BEST COOK   ix

CHAPTER 1:   COOK YOUR WAY TO A GREAT BODY   3

CHAPTER 2:   THE CALORIE-CYCLING KITCHEN   13

CHAPTER 3:   FAST-FUEL MEALS   23

    FAST-FUEL BREAKFASTS   24

    FAST-FUEL LUNCHES   34

    FAST-FUEL DINNERS   58

    FAST-FUEL SNACKS   92

CHAPTER 4:   SLOW-FUEL MEALS   97

    SLOW-FUEL BREAKFASTS   98

    SLOW-FUEL LUNCHES   107

    SLOW-FUEL DINNERS   124

    SLOW-FUEL SNACKS   149

CHAPTER 5:   SMOOTHIES AND JUICES   153

CHAPTER 6:   FAST-FUEL DESSERTS   181

CHAPTER 7:   BLOCK OUT YOUR MEALS   195

    SAMPLE BLOCK 3 MENUS   199

    SAMPLE BLOCK 2 MENUS   217

    SAMPLE BLOCK 1 MENUS   229

    SAMPLE PLANT-BASED MENUS   236

ACKNOWLEDGMENTS   255

REFERENCES   257

INDEX   259

INTRODUCTION

YOU ARE YOUR OWN BEST COOK

Just as your body is your own gym—the greatest fitness machine ever—you are your own best cook. You don't have to rely on pop-in-the-microwave junk food, grab-and-go fast food, or other less-than-healthful meal solutions. I've created this cookbook for people who want to gain muscle, lose fat, improve performance and energy, stay healthy, or all of the above. The recipes I offer you in this cookbook—as well as the shopping lists and meal plans—reflect the way that I eat when I cook for myself. If you have read my book *You Are Your Own Gym*, you know that I am a fan of do-it-yourself exercise. If you have read my book *Body Fuel*, you know that I have a specific strategy for eating that keeps your metabolism guessing and promotes a lean and well-defined physique. This cookbook supports both my workout programs and my eating strategies. It's just what you need to start preparing delicious home-style meals, lean and tasty comfort foods, spicy regional favorites, international entrées, even desserts—all with the end result in mind: a lean, defined body.

Sound good so far?

Great! One of the real secrets of weight and fitness management is cooking at home more often than going out to eat. You get to control the content and quality of your food, make better choices about what and how much you eat, plus take charge of your physique and how it looks.

You see, restaurant food is notoriously high in salt, fat, sugar, and additives—that's what makes it taste so good. But that's also what makes fat creep on, especially if you habitually eat in restaurants. Am I saying never eat out? Absolutely not—that would be unrealistic. But when you don't control the preparation of your own food, who knows what hidden fats, sodium, sugars, and additives are lurking in the food you're consuming? It's okay to dine out once in a while, but be reasonable, and be conscious about putting whole, clean, and preferably organic foods into your body. These foods contain the nutrients you need to strengthen your body, transform your physique, and promote a youthful, energetic appearance.

And it's not only me who thinks that eating more meals at home results in a more healthful diet. According to recent research reported in the journal *Public Health Nutrition*, more frequent cooking at home was associated with eating a more healthful diet and consuming less fat, sugar, carbohydrates, and overall calories. And understandably, more frequent cooking at home was associated with consuming fewer calories away from home and eating less fast food. These findings are certainly "food for thought" if you want to change the way you look and feel.

Don't get me wrong—I've certainly done my fair share of eating out and eating on the road. And that's to your benefit in the end: I've become familiar with the wonderful flavors and textures of many different types of cuisines. At home, I've obsessively sandpapered down the fat, sugar, and calories to create lighter versions of my favorite comfort foods (macaroni and cheese, chow mein, milkshakes, cupcakes, and more!) so that I can eat delicious food that also supports my physical training and helps accentuate muscular development and definition.

Through this experience, my love affair with cooking was born, and it's only grown deeper with more time spent in the kitchen. Whether experimenting with recipes by myself or cooking for my friends or loved ones, I'm never more satisfied than when I have a spatula or spoon in my hand.

Although I'd love for you to believe that I'm a culinary genius, the more I cook, the more I realize anyone can do it. My recipes are very basic and quick to prepare. (And after serving in the Special Forces, I can say with confidence that they sure beat military chow.) Anyway, can you read? Can you follow easy instructions? Of course you can—and that means you can cook! Get started!

YOU ARE YOUR OWN GYM
THE COOKBOOK

Protein

+

FAST FUEL

+

SLOW FUEL

Protein

+

FAST FUEL

Protein

+

SLOW FUEL

Protein

+

FAST FUEL

+

SLOW FUEL

Chapter 1

Cook Your Way to a Great Body

With this cookbook, you'll be creating delicious meals that support my secret weapon for fat loss and muscle building, which I introduced in *Body Fuel:* calorie cycling. Unlike the typical calorie-restrictive diet, in which you stick to a static, low-calorie plan, calorie cycling periodically changes your caloric intake, up or down; your calories never stay constant for more than a few weeks. By jerking your metabolism around so that it never gets sluggish but keeps burning fat, calorie cycling naturally leads to more body-firming muscle and less unsightly (and unhealthful) fat. This concept is similar to what happens when you change your workout volume and intensity from time to time in order to keep your body adapting to new stimuli. Periodic changes in your caloric intake (volume) and strictness of your fuel choices (intensity) do the same thing. Calorie cycling leads to more muscle and less fat than if you were to follow the same diet for four weeks straight or longer.

Calorie cycling also prevents diet plateauing, in which you seem to stop losing weight, or you find that your clothes aren't getting looser anymore. You're stuck. Every serious athlete, exerciser, or dieter has been there and done that. With calorie cycling, there's less likelihood of plateauing until you have reached your target weight, because there's more change, and that equals more adaptation.

On my plan, you're also encouraged to eat a wider range of foods than most weight-loss diets prescribe. That's because many of the foods (such as fruit and other carbs) normally restricted on diets purely about weight loss are actually required for building muscle and recovering from good, hard workouts.

FAST FUEL, SLOW FUEL

When you are calorie-cycling, the adjustment of calories—up or down—comes primarily from the carbohydrates you choose. I look at carbs as "slow" or "fast" based on the speed at which the body absorbs them.

All carbohydrates must be converted to glucose, a type of sugar, before they are absorbed into the bloodstream. Carbs are absorbed at either a fast rate or a slow rate. That rate of absorption produces a proportionately strong release of the hormone insulin, which regulates the amount of sugar in the blood. When we eat carbs that absorb *quickly* (fast-fuel carbs), such as candy, soda, fruit, or fruit juice, an insulin surge rapidly depletes blood sugar and converts these carbs to fat. We're also left feeling tired, and we crave more food to restore normal blood sugar levels. There's a positive exception to this scenario, though: eating some fast-fuel carbs during or immediately after intense exercise replenishes depleted muscles and aids in the recovery and building process.

By contrast, slow-fuel carbs such as vegetables are absorbed more slowly and do not produce this fat-gaining insulin reaction. Slow-fuel carbs also tend to be lower in calories, high in fat-burning fiber, and packed with many more vitamins and minerals than some fast-fuel carbs.

GLYCEMIC INDEX VERSUS GLYCEMIC LOAD

How can you tell which carbs are fast-fuel and which are slow-fuel?

I use a tool called the *glycemic load*, or GL. GL is a numerical ranking system for carbs that measures the amount of carbohydrates in a standard serving of food, say a banana or a cup of rice, and how fast or slow the carbohydrates in that food are released into the bloodstream. The GL number is the best indicator of what a particular food does to your blood sugar. The lower the GL of a food, the better it is for weight control and overall health.

Now, you might be thinking: "Is glycemic load the same as glycemic index?" No. The glycemic index indicates how quickly a carb turns into sugar in your bloodstream, but it does not consider how much carbohydrate there is in a particular serving—in other words, the amount you actually eat. It's better to focus on the glycemic load instead.

SLOW-FUEL CARBS

Slow-fuel carbs have a GL rating of 1 to 6, and they include all low-calorie, high-fiber vegetables such as greens, salad vegetables, broccoli, cauliflower, green beans, tomatoes, yellow squash, zucchini, and so forth. These can be eaten with reckless abandon at any time. At most of your meals every day, you want to include slow-fuel carbs.

Slow-fuel carbs are also low in calories and high in fiber—properties that fight weight gain and promote weight control. You can fill up on slow-fuel carbs because their calorie counts are negligible. You stay full longer and can resist the "urge to splurge" on fattening foods. Plus, the fiber in slow-fuel carbs is a true anti-obesity weapon. The less processed and the more natural the food (like slow-fuel carbs), the fewer calories and less fat your body absorbs. The fiber also keeps you feeling full, so you don't overeat.

FAST-FUEL CARBS

Carbs with a GL of 7 or higher—including healthful options such as grains, grain-based products, potatoes, pasta, sweet potatoes, rice, and fruit, and much less healthful options such as fruit juice, sports drinks, and sodas—are considered fast-fuel carbs. They stimulate a greater insulin release and are digested and absorbed quickly by the body.

There are two specific times of day that it's okay to eat fast carbs: upon waking in the morning and after a rigorous workout.

Overnight sleep is effectively a fast. This overnight fast depletes glycogen—the carbohydrate stored in your muscles and liver. Unless you break the fast, your body will start breaking down muscle tissue for fuel—a bad scenario if you're trying to develop muscle or burn fat. Eating a fast-fuel carb shortly after you awaken will crank out insulin and rapidly replenish your glycogen levels to halt the possible assault on your muscles.

Fast-fuel carbs quickly restock glycogen after exercise as well. Right after you exercise and up to about forty-five minutes thereafter, your blood flow is elevated, so any carbs you eat will get into your system rapidly. Your muscles and liver are more receptive to insulin at this time, so insulin can get to work to restock glycogen in your muscles. Other enzymes and hormones active in muscle repair and growth have peaked at this time as well. If you delay eating after exercise—say, for a couple of hours or longer—these enzymes and hormones fall by nearly two-thirds and keep falling from there, and your body quickly moves from an anabolic state (building muscle) to a catabolic state (cannibalizing muscle for protein and fuel). So don't miss this important window of metabolic opportunity. Good post-workout refueling choices include brown rice, whole-grain bread, pasta, potatoes, fresh juice, or smoothies. So remember, if you're active and training hard, it's okay—indeed, it's a good idea—to include fast-fuel carbs in your diet, especially if you're trying to gain strength and build muscle mass.

PROTEIN FUEL

In addition to slow- and fast-fuel carbs, you'll want to eat ample protein. Beef, lamb, pork, poultry, fish, eggs, tofu, and beans all supply protein. If you don't eat enough protein, your metabolism can slow down. Muscle is metabolic tissue that requires calories, so if your body dismantles muscle to fulfill its protein requirements, you're losing a key factor in fat burning.

Protein drives your muscle development and fat-burning mechanisms, particularly when coupled with regular exercise. After you eat protein, it's broken down into amino acids, the building blocks used to repair and regenerate all cells. One of these amino acids is called leucine, and it seems to be the best of the bunch. Your muscles use it as fuel. It helps you develop and maintain lean muscle mass, enabling your body to burn more calories for a boost in weight loss. Animal-based proteins are very high in leucine.

Protein activates your body's fat-burning mechanisms in another way: by helping to produce a hormone called glucagon. Glucagon is like an instant message to your body, directing it to move dietary fat out of storage into your bloodstream, where it can be burned for fuel.

Protein helps you feel full, too, by boosting levels of a hormone called peptide YY, which is obviously of benefit when you're restricting food to lose weight. When you're thinking about wolfing down some sweets or you're craving carbs, eat a small bite of protein instead. More than likely your hunger will disappear.

There are other benefits to eating protein. The energy (calories) from protein is used to develop and repair all the body's tissues, especially the muscles. Proteins regulate your body's water balance. Protein is also key to the manufacture of red blood cells, enzymes, hormones, and antibodies that are essential for the proper functioning of your body.

HOW MUCH PROTEIN?

I advise eating 3 to 6 ounces of protein foods with every main meal. That amount of food approximates the size of your fist. So play up protein—and watch your body change for the better.

FAT FUEL

If you've read *You Are Your Own Gym*, *Body by You*, or *Body Fuel*, you will already know that my fitness and eating goals are to maximize lean body mass and minimize body fat. It might surprise you to learn that the typical low-fat diet will not accomplish this; you actually need to eat a diet slightly higher in fat.

The current word on this comes from a study published in September 2014 in the *Annals of Internal Medicine*. Researchers assigned a group of 150 men and women to follow a diet for one year that was low-carb (fewer than 40 grams of carbs daily) and either higher in fat or low in fat.

It turned out that the low-carb/higher-fat dieters lost about eight pounds more on average than those on the low-fat diet. The low-carb/higher fat dieters had significantly greater reductions in body fat, too, as well as improvements in lean muscle mass, even though neither group changed their exercise level. In fact, the weight lost by the low-fat dieters was mostly muscle mass. I was encouraged after reading these results, since my way of eating gives me a bit more fat than most diets.

There are two general types of dietary fat: saturated and unsaturated. Saturated fat comes mainly from animal sources as well as from coconut oil. Unsaturated fats are derived mainly from plant sources such as nuts, seeds, avocados, olive oil, and flaxseed oil, as well as from fish.

Eating some saturated fat is vital for active people because it helps maintain concentrations of testosterone circulating in the body. Testosterone helps develop muscle and promote strength. Research has shown that men who get less than 30 percent of their calories from fat produce 25 percent less testosterone than those who have more fat in their diets.

Don't get me wrong: I'm not advocating that you go out and start packing away bacon, butter, and marbled rib-eyes like there's no tomorrow. Too much of any nutrient is bad for you, especially when it's out of proportion to other vital nutrients. Balance is key.

HOW MUCH FAT?

Fat makes up 25 to 35 percent of my total calorie intake. That fat comes from both saturated and unsaturated sources. You'll naturally get the right balance of fats if you eat a small palmful of nuts and seeds, add 1 tablespoon of oil (olive, flaxseed, or coconut) to your daily diet, and consume animal sources of protein.

If you're a vegetarian or a vegan, using coconut oil in the diet will provide you with some needed saturated fat.

CALORIE CYCLING AND FUEL BLOCKS

When you calorie-cycle, you will follow three eating "blocks," each with differing amounts of carbs and calories. Think of the blocks in descending numerical order—3, 2, 1—and as blocks that last as long as their label. This system is easy to remember and easy to incorporate into your lifestyle, but the most important thing to under-stand is that cycling through the blocks is something you can customize and keep doing and doing and doing. You can eat this way for the rest of your life. Your body and metabolism won't become accustomed to the same old eating patterns—which lead to weight loss plateaus or ruts—but instead will continuously be tricked and triggered so that you continue to burn fuel efficiently and stay lean and strong, even after you've reached your goal weight or clothing size. Same blocks, but a fooled body every time.

BLOCK 3

The first block is the most liberal phase of the diet, and happily for you, it lasts the longest: three weeks, which is why I call it Block 3. You can have a lot of the fast-fuel carbs you love—one serving at each meal and one snack, for a total of four carbs daily. Think bread, pasta, potatoes, rice, and all sorts of fruit. Can you believe it? Don't worry: you can lose a chunk of weight by eating these fuels. You can build more body-firming muscle and recover much more quickly after your workouts. And you won't even feel like you're dieting. You get to eat on Block 3 (in fact, you have to, in order to create the body you want) without continuously restricting calories. It's a dream: the return of good food, which is absolutely necessary in the right doses for the development of an athletic, fat-burning body.

After three weeks of that, you'll be noticeably trimmer. The scale will register a big drop in weight. The mirror will show a fitter you. Your clothes will fit better; in fact, you may have to go shopping for a smaller size. And you'll feel more energetic, simply by making realistic, sustainable, and important dietary changes. But so that you don't plateau, you've got to change up your metabolism—which requires switching to Block 2 after three weeks.

Worth mentioning here: Once you've achieved your fitness goals, use Block 3 to maintain your weight and stay in shape.

MEAL DESIGN FOR BLOCK 3

Breakfast Pattern: protein + 1 serving fast-fuel carb
Lunch Pattern: protein + 1 serving fast-fuel carb and liberal amounts of slow-fuel carbs
Dinner Pattern: protein + 1 serving fast-fuel carb and liberal amounts of slow-fuel carbs
Snack Pattern (1 midmorning, 1 midafternoon): protein + nuts or seeds or a slow-fuel carb; as your second snack have a protein + a fast-fuel carb. This pattern should be eaten following a workout.

BLOCK 2

Block 2 comes next and, you guessed it, lasts two weeks. During this block, you'll continue to eat most of the same foods, but with one exception: you'll reduce your carbs slightly, to two fast-fuel carbs a day. Overall, Block 2 is a little less liberal than Block 3, food-wise, but it keeps you in a fat-burning mode, so you can taper down to your ideal weight.

MEAL DESIGN FOR BLOCK 2

Breakfast Pattern: protein + 1 fast-fuel carb

Lunch Pattern: protein + 1 fast-fuel carb + slow-fuel carbs

Dinner Pattern: protein + slow-fuel carbs

Snack Pattern (1 midmorning, 1 midafternoon): protein + nuts or seeds or a slow-fuel carb (or, after a workout, protein + a fast-fuel carb, if not eaten at one of your three main meals)

BLOCK 1

Block 1 lasts for one week and is the most restrictive of the blocks. But remember, it's only one week, and then you go back to the top with Block 3 to eat more liberally. In Block 1, you'll cut your fast-fuel carbs down to one carb a day. Don't panic: anyone can do anything if it's just for seven days. You'll be amazed at how well you'll breeze through this week. The weight loss you've experienced up to this point will motivate you to tighten up your food choices, and you won't miss those extra carbs one bit. Even if you find Block 1 easy, it's important to cycle back to the eating style of Block 3 thereafter, especially if you're engaged in intense physical activity.

MEAL DESIGN FOR BLOCK 1

Breakfast Pattern: protein + 1 fast-fuel carb or 1 slow-fuel carb

Lunch Pattern: protein + slow-fuel carb

Dinner Pattern: protein + slow-fuel carb

Snack Pattern (1 midmorning, 1 midafternoon): protein + nuts or seeds or a slow-fuel carb (or, after a workout, protein + a slow-fuel carb, if not eaten at one of your three main meals)

CALORIE CYCLING AT A GLANCE

BLOCK 3 (3 weeks): 4 fast-fuel carbs daily and liberal amounts of slow-fuel carbs	
Breakfast	Protein + 1 fast-fuel carb
Lunch	Protein + 1 fast-fuel carb + slow-fuel carbs
Dinner	Protein + 1 fast-fuel carb + slow-fuel carbs
Snack 1	Protein + nuts or seeds or a slow-fuel carb
Snack 2	Protein + fast-fuel carbs (Have this snack pattern after a workout.)
BLOCK 2 (2 weeks): 2 fast-fuel carbs daily and liberal amounts of slow-fuel carbs	
Breakfast	Protein + 1 fast-fuel carb
Lunch	Protein + 1 fast-fuel carb + slow-fuel carbs
Dinner	Protein + slow-fuel carbs
Snack 1	Protein + nuts or seeds or a slow-fuel carb
Snack 2	Protein + slow-fuel carbs (or, after a workout, protein + 1 fast-fuel carb, if not eaten at one of your three main meals)
BLOCK 1 (1 week): 1 fast-fuel carb daily and liberal amounts of slow-fuel carbs	
Breakfast	Protein + 1 fast-fuel carb or 1 slow-fuel carb
Lunch	Protein + slow-fuel carbs
Dinner	Protein + slow-fuel carbs
Snack 1	Protein + slow-fuel carbs
Snack 2	Protein + slow-fuel carbs (or, after a workout, protein + fast-fuel carb, if not eaten at one of your three main meals)

USING THIS COOKBOOK

To make it easy to choose foods and recipes to meet your calorie-cycling needs, I've divided the recipes in this cookbook into chapters corresponding to my fast-fuel, slow-fuel eating system. My recipes also follow four rules: they are easy to fix, intensely flavored, made with the freshest and best ingredients possible, and quick to prepare. And for anyone watching a food budget, I like to offer recipes that are affordable and won't break the household bank.

As a very useful addition, each of the recipes has its nutritional content listed, including calories per portion, in case you like to count those. My hope is to provide you with delicious and nutritious recipes that will satisfy your palate and keep you on the right track. All the recipes are so simple that you can whip them up even if you have no previous cooking experience. The sample meal plans show you how to build your daily menus with the recipes, too.

In addition, each recipe serving is a complete meal, with protein, vegetables, and more. (There are vegetarian and vegan recipes here, too; the vegan recipes are marked by a V.) Feel free to adjust your portions up or down. If you are intent on losing weight, you'll want to eat the recommended portion or slightly less. On the other hand, if you want to put on mass or want to maintain your weight, eat a slightly larger portion.

Each recipe makes anywhere from 1 serving to a meal for 6 or more. I actually find that making multiple servings—a whole casserole dish of a dinner or a whole tin of breakfast muffins—helps me stick to my eating objectives because when I am short on time, I have healthful leftovers to choose from. If you operate the same way, feel free to double or triple a recipe so that you have extra in the fridge. Obviously, you can also reduce the recipe to fewer servings, if you know that having leftovers around might tempt you to overeat.

My recipes are based on *real fuel*, those foods closest to what our ancient ancestors ate, including meats, fish, vegetables, fruit, grains, nuts, and seeds—essentially natural, power-packed food—put together in a diet that is most compatible with our genetic makeup. Millions of years ago, people who ate these foods and used them to fuel their physically demanding lives were the fittest of the species, the survivors. Eating whole foods is the reason we can perform at our best—and look our best.

If you're new to home cooking, try at least three or four of these recipes the first week. Keep trying a couple of new recipes each week after that. Eventually I want you to use this cookbook all the time, rather than just opening it sporadically. Think of this as an adventure. I love adventure, because it's fun. And you'll have fun trying new dishes.

So follow me—some tasty bites are just a few pages away.

Chapter 2

The Calorie-Cycling Kitchen

Come to my house, and on any given day you'll find my pantry and fridge overflowing with every "body fuel" imaginable, from lean proteins to veggies to fruits, plus all sorts of condiments, nuts, and spices. With the right ingredients on hand, I can whip up a meal that fits my block needs without much forethought.

As you prepare to calorie-cycle through the three-block system, I'd suggest a pantry and fridge renovation. By this, I mean throw out any junk food. Just about anything that comes in a box (with the exception of whole grains) or enveloped in a candy wrapper is junk food. It's normally loaded with sugar, trans fats, and preservatives. If you eat more sugar, fat, and other junk than you burn off, your body generates fat. Globs of sunny yellow fat—unused glucose that's now turned to fat—float in your blood through your arteries to organs or tissues, where they are deposited. When fat finds a home somewhere, you get fat and look fat. That's the cosmetic problem we all hate and want to do away with. Also critical: when fat homesteads in an organ, it can cause big problems, from heart disease to diabetes to outright organ failure. So junk the junk—and be brutal about it.

After the pantry and fridge purge, it's time to restock. You don't have to do this all at once; just base it on what you're going to require for the week ahead. Here are some basic guidelines for stocking up on staples that will make meal planning and preparation much easier—and more healthful.

GRASS-FED MEATS AND FREE-RANGE POULTRY

It's important to consider the methods used to grow or raise our food and also the processes used to get that food onto our plates, because ultimately the health of the livestock we eat affects our health. For this reason, I'm conscious and cautious about whether the poultry I eat is free-range, meaning the birds have been allowed to roam freely outdoors and eat whatever grass, seeds, or insects they choose. I also make sure they have not been given hormones or antibiotics. This results in more nutritious poultry and is more humane to the animals. I'm also concerned whether the meat I eat is grass-fed rather than grain-fed. With the exception of the mother cow's milk before weaning, this means that the cattle were raised entirely eating grass from pastures, as opposed to being fed with grain. Why is grass-fed better? Meat from grass-fed livestock:

• Has fewer calories
• Is packed with more vitamin E, beta-carotene, and vitamin C

- Is richer in omega-3 fatty acids
- Contains a higher concentration of conjugated linoleic acid, or CLA—a "good" fat that may strengthen immunity, normalize blood sugar, and help fat burning in the body
- Is unlikely to contain any additives, including chemicals, pesticides, growth hormones, or genetically modified feed

It's also smart to shop for meat that is labeled "organic." Animals raised organically have not been given hormones or antibiotics to promote growth. Although they may have eaten only organic feed, they may not be grass-fed, however. When you're shopping for healthful poultry and meat, the best choice is to look for the "certified organic" and "grass-fed" or "free-range" labels.

SALMON AND OTHER SEAFOOD

Fish is an excellent source of protein, too, and it's also loaded with omega-3 fatty acids. These amazing fats have the power to affect fat metabolism, diverting it away from storage and burning it for energy. If your belly runneth over, eat fish, particularly salmon and tuna. Both are high in omega-3 fats, known to help reduce abdominal fat. Wild-caught fish is best because it's typically not laced with antibiotics, dyes, and artificial growth promoters. You can also check out the website seafoodwatch.org for a list of sustainably harvested fish, plus seafood that is lowest in toxins.

EGGS

Eggs have been nicknamed the "perfect food." They are a source of high-quality protein and contain a number of vitamins and minerals. Eggs also have an extremely high biological value, which means that the body absorbs and retains egg protein completely and efficiently. Plus, they have been shown to help control appetite. Choose eggs from free-range chickens that aren't fed hormones or antibiotics.

PROTEIN POWDERS

My smoothie and juice recipes call for the addition of protein powder. Whey-based protein powders are a good choice, especially since whey has been associated with fat burning and muscle building. You may want to choose a plant-based protein powder, however. There are several guidelines to bear in mind when choosing plant-based protein powders. First, look at the label. The very first ingredient should be the vegetable protein source. Typically, other protein powders might list some form of non-vegetable protein, or milk or egg proteins. Second, read the label again to make sure that it's free of genetically modified ingredients (GMOs), sugar, fructose, and any artificial flavor.

I don't recommend that you choose a protein powder made with soy. Soy can mess with your hormonal balance over time and isn't good for weight control. Finally, an organic blend is a healthful choice when you're looking at different brands.

VEGETABLES

My recipes are heavy on vegetables—both slow-fuel veggies (low in calories, high in fiber) and fast-fuel veggies (those slightly higher in starch, such as potatoes and sweet potatoes). Although canned or frozen vegetables are convenient, fresh produce is always a better choice when you have time to prepare it. The less time that elapses between field and market, the more flavor and nutrients the products retain. If possible, choose organically grown over picture-perfect produce that may be sprayed with chemicals and waxes.

FRUITS

My recipes also use all sorts of fruits, from fresh to dried. Fruits tend to be high in fiber, which means the body digests them more slowly, and that makes for better hunger management and weight control than other sources of sweet, simple sugars. Plus, fruit is loaded with antioxidants and other natural substances that keep your body in peak health.

Unlike slow-fuel vegetables, though, fruit is not a free food. Fruit still falls under the umbrella of carbs that must be controlled. Fruit is a fast fuel.

The other thing I advise people about fruit is the risk associated with pesticides. If you're eating fruit that doesn't have a thick peel, such as an apple or berries, buy organic and wash them well. Fruits that do have thick peels, such as citrus and bananas, are pretty well protected by the peels themselves, so I don't think you need to spend the extra money on organic.

BREADS, GRAINS, CEREALS, AND PASTA

Too often we generalize and wind up labeling an entire category of food as being "bad." Carbs are definitely one of those categories that have gotten a bad rap. They are not all the same, and it's important that you distinguish between good carbs and lesser ones.

For example, if a piece of bread can be turned into a ball of dough simply by squeezing it in your hand, it should probably be avoided unless you're looking for a quick post-workout sugar and insulin boost to replenish lost glycogen stores. Here's why: to make such a fine-grained white product, the bran (hard outer shell) and the germ (reproductive part) of whole grains are removed during a mechanical grinding process, leaving only the fast-absorbed sugars. This process also takes out most of the vitamins and fiber. Bleach and other chemicals are often then added to further soften and whiten the grain.

These highly refined and processed grains are what make up the bulk of grain products found packaged in grocery stores, and they are largely responsible for our weight and health problems. But this does not make all grain products bad, especially if you're fairly active and exercise regularly! You'll want to include the more healthful, far less processed grain choices in your diet to fuel hard workouts and to help you recover properly, so you can get the most possible benefit from every squat, lunge, press, and pull. Don't go completely grain-dead on me: making smart grain selections is easy. If you're cutting out gluten, choose gluten-free grains.

FAST-FUEL GRAIN-BASED FOODS FOR YOUR PANTRY

Brown rice	Whole-grain bread
Edamame spaghetti	Whole-grain flatbreads
Kelp noodles	Whole-wheat orzo
Oatmeal	Whole-wheat pasta
Panko (Japanese-style bread crumbs)	Whole-wheat pita breads
Quinoa	Whole-wheat tortillas
Soba (buckwheat) noodles	Wild rice

SWEETENERS

My recipes call for various types of sweeteners, but in very tiny amounts. And none of my recipes use artificial sweeteners, which can make you fat—even the occasional diet soda. Fake sweeteners cause many of the same reactions that regular sugar does, because the receptors on your tongue and in your stomach can't discern between real sugar and fake sugar. So artificial sweeteners only trick the brain into craving more sweets and more sugar and throw your blood sugar levels out of balance. Also, our bodies weren't designed to process artificial ingredients, and they do no favors to your body.

SWEETENERS FOR YOUR PANTRY

Agave syrup

Brown sugar

Granulated sugar

Honey

NUTS AND SEEDS

I'm a big fan of nuts and seeds, and I use them in many of my recipes. High in unsaturated fats, nuts and seeds are packed with fiber, protein, and beneficial antioxidants. They're also brimming with glutamine, an amino acid that helps spare lean muscle. Nuts and seeds are good appetite regulators, too. (Just don't stuff yourself with them, because they are very high in calories.)

NUTS AND SEEDS FOR YOUR PANTRY

Almonds

Chia seeds

Coconut, unsweetened shredded

Flaxseed

Hemp seeds

Peanuts

Pine nuts

Pumpkin seeds

Sesame seeds

Sunflower seeds

Walnuts

DAIRY AND NON-DAIRY FOODS

Dairy is used only in minuscule amounts in my recipes, and only as a way to impart a smooth, creamy quality to certain dishes. I generally limit dairy foods because they produce high insulin responses, despite being low-glycemic foods. This is because dairy foods contain lactose, a sugar (unless they are formulated to be lactose-free).

As for full-fat dairy foods, many people avoid them because they believe such foods will make them fat. That thinking, however, defies the results of a large study published in the *European Journal of Nutrition* in 2013 which found that high-fat dairy was associated with a lower risk of obesity. But why? Some researchers point to the satiety factor. The higher fat in dairy foods may make us feel fuller faster, and thus we may end up eating less.

Others believe there may be bioactive substances in milk fat that may alter our metabolism in ways that help us burn more fat for energy, rather than store it in our bodies. Even so, many of my recipes sidestep dairy altogether and use tasty substitutes such as almond milk or coconut milk.

DAIRY FOR YOUR FRIDGE

Fat-free cottage cheese

Fat-free mozzarella

Fat-free plain yogurt

Feta cheese, low-fat and regular

Goat cheese

Half-and-half

Low-fat cheeses

Low-fat Greek yogurt

Low-fat milk

Non-dairy milks: almond milk, coconut milk

Parmesan cheese

Parmigiano-Reggiano cheese

Pecorino Romano cheese

Queso fresco

Skim milk

Smoked Gouda

Swiss cheese

BUTTER AND OILS

I recommend that you consume 1 tablespoon daily of either olive oil, flaxseed oil, or coconut oil (the last of these is a plant source of saturated fat). These are advantageous because, instead of being easily packed on as body fat, they enhance muscle growth and fat burning. Many of my recipes use these oils, so be sure to count the oil in your daily allotment. Some recipes call for a little butter—a saturated fat that is actually good for you in moderation because it supports healthy hormone production in the body.

BUTTER AND OILS FOR YOUR PANTRY AND FRIDGE

Almond butter

Avocado oil

Butter

Coconut oil

Cooking spray

Flaxseed oil

Olive oil

Sesame oil

HERBS AND SPICES

Herbs and spices jazz up any recipe. If you fancy Indian, try a little turmeric. Chinese? Add in some ginger. Mexican? Bring on the cumin. Buy small quantities, as herbs and spices lose flavor intensity over time. Buy fresh herbs when a recipe calls for them. Keep dried seasonings in tightly closed jars away from heat and light.

HERBS AND SPICES FOR YOUR PANTRY

Bay leaves

Black pepper

Cayenne

Chili powder

Cinnamon

Cloves, ground

Coriander seeds

Creole seasoning

Crushed red pepper

Cumin, ground

Curry powder

Dill, dried

Fennel seeds

Five-spice powder (an Asian spice blend)

Garam masala

Garlic powder

Italian seasoning

Mustard, dry

Nutmeg

Onion powder

Oregano, dried

Paprika

Peppercorns

Rosemary, dried

Salt (table salt, kosher salt, or
  coarse Himalayan salt)

Thyme, dried

White pepper

MISCELLANEOUS

Baking powder

Capers

Cornstarch

Low-fat, low-sodium chicken broth

Low-fat, low-sodium vegetable broth

Vanilla extract

Worcestershire sauce

CONDIMENTS

I like to flavor my recipes with an assortment of condiments. They're pretty low in calories and they make sticking to a calorie-cycling lifestyle very easy. Like herbs and spices, these savory substances complement the natural taste of foods and can transform uninspired dishes into memorable ones. Stock up on the following:

Apple cider vinegar

Barbecue sauce

Brown mustard, whole-grain and regular

Cholula Hot Sauce

Dijon mustard

Fish sauce

Low-fat mayonnaise

Low-sodium soy sauce

Low-sugar or low-carbohydrate pasta sauce

Miso

Ponzu (Japanese citrus-based sauce)

Red wine vinegar

Sriracha

Thai green curry paste

White vinegar

White wine vinegar

Wasabi

KITCHEN EQUIPMENT

In my workout courses, I advocate a no-equipment approach to exercising. None of my workouts require any fancy equipment, daunting machines, or weird contraptions or gadgets to squeeze. You employ the best workout "machine" ever designed: your body. Using your body's own resistance, you can develop greater strength, power, muscular and cardiovascular endurance, tone, and definition than you ever thought possible.

It's a slightly different story when cooking up my meals, though. You do need equipment to make meal magic! That said, most of what you need is probably already in your kitchen:

MEASURING TOOLS

Measuring spoons

Measuring cups

POTS AND PANS

Skillets, various sizes

Large ovenproof nonstick skillet

Pots, various sizes

Baking sheet

Baking dish (9 by 13 inches)

Baking pan (9 inches square)

9-inch pie plate

12-cup muffin tin

Round cake pan

Shallow serving dish

Wok

UTENSILS

Whisks

Mixing spoons

Large fork

Salad tongs

Spatulas

Kitchen knives, various sizes

SMALL APPLIANCES

Blender

Juicer

Food processor

Spiralizer

Slow cooker, 4-quart

Microwave

Outdoor grill

OTHER HELPFUL ITEMS

Mixing bowls, various sizes

Cutting boards, various sizes

Colander

Grater

Plastic kitchen bags for marinating

8-inch skewers

Small mason jars or containers

Chapter 3

Fast-Fuel Meals

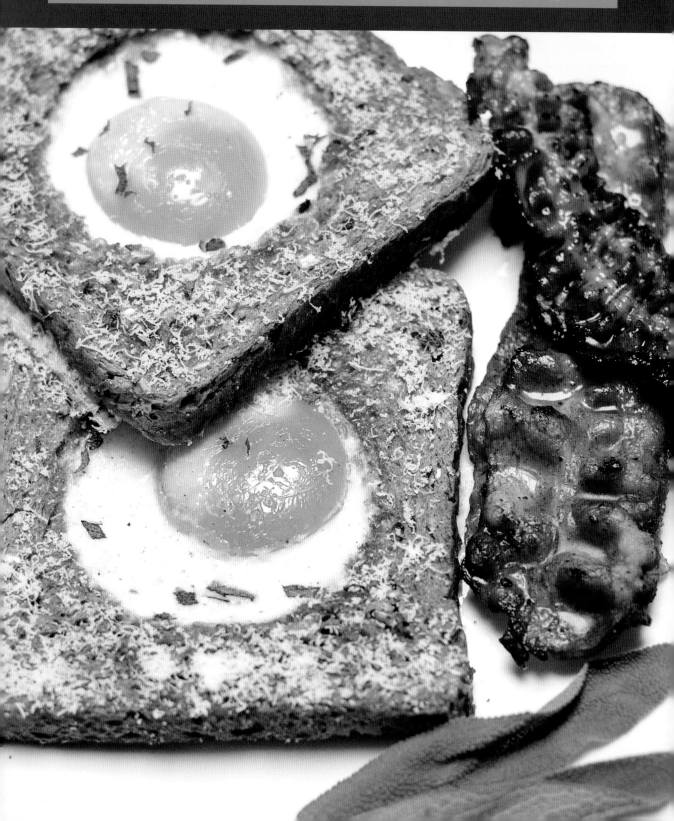

BAKED EGG IN A HOLE

Experts agree that breakfast is the most important meal of the day, but eating the same predictable dishes over and over can make this essential meal a very boring one. Instead, start off your day with this twist on the traditional bacon-and-eggs breakfast. No need to worry about the saturated fat in bacon, either. The verdict from new research is that there's no significant proof that dietary saturated fat is linked to an increased risk for heart disease. The fast fuel in this breakfast is the whole-wheat bread.

1 SERVING

1 slice bacon

1 slice whole-wheat bread, lightly toasted

1 large egg

1 teaspoon grated Parmesan cheese

1/4 teaspoon chopped fresh sage

1/4 teaspoon garlic powder

Preheat oven to 400 degrees.

Cook the bacon over medium heat in a small skillet until crisp; drain on paper towels.

Cut a hole in the center of the toast using a small juice glass or a round cookie cutter. Reserve the cutout.

Coat a baking sheet with cooking spray. Arrange bread slice (and center cutout) on pan and crack the egg into the hole. Sprinkle with cheese, sage, and garlic powder. Season with salt and pepper. Bake for 5 minutes or until egg white is set. Serve with bacon and toast cutout.

NUTRITION PER SERVING | FAT: 10 GRAMS | CARBOHYDRATE: 14 GRAMS | PROTEIN: 13 GRAMS | TOTAL CALORIES: 198

COMPLETE MORNING GLORY

The American Dietetic Association reports that people who skip breakfast tend to gain, on average, one pound a week because they overcompensate by overeating later in the morning and at lunch. I know you don't want that, so here's a complete meal full of nutrients, protein, and fast fuel in the form of whole-wheat bread and berries that will curb your hunger all morning long. Don't be a skipper!

1 SERVING

4 turkey sausage links
1 large egg
1/2 cup blueberries

1/2 cup sliced strawberries
1 slice whole-wheat bread, toasted

Heat a skillet over medium heat and sauté sausage until cooked through; set aside.

Coat the same skillet with cooking spray. Crack the egg into the skillet. Cook until the egg white is set.

While the egg is cooking, mix the blueberries and strawberries together to make a side of fruit.

Serve berries with sausage, egg, and toast.

NUTRITION PER SERVING | FAT: 14 GRAMS | CARBOHYDRATE: 20 GRAMS | PROTEIN: 20 GRAMS | TOTAL CALORIES: 286

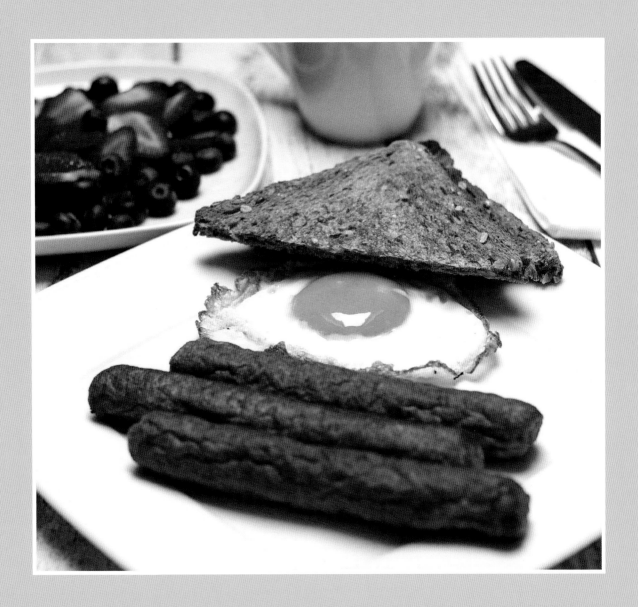

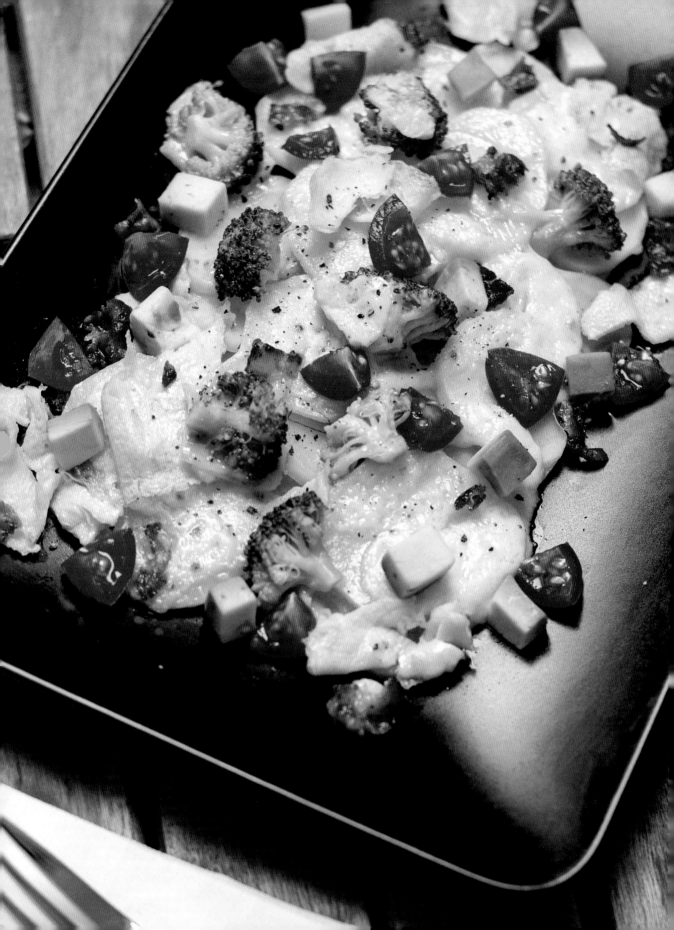

BAKED POTATOES WITH EGGS

I'm a bit of a breakfast freak, especially if the first meal of the day has all the food groups joined together and tastes amazing, as this one does. In fact, this recipe is one of my favorites. It's got protein, potatoes, lots of veggies, cheese, and a bacon-y flavor—everything you need to energize the rest of your day. Since it requires a little more time to prepare than some of my other breakfasts, I like to make multiple servings at once. Just refrigerate what you aren't eating today.

8 SERVINGS

1 tablespoon olive oil

1/2 cup finely chopped yellow onions

11/2 cups low-fat milk

4 teaspoons all-purpose flour

1/2 teaspoon salt

1/4 teaspoon black pepper

1 cup shredded reduced-fat sharp cheddar cheese

6 russet or white potatoes, peeled and sliced

11/2 cups chopped broccoli

4 large eggs

4 egg whites

6 slices turkey bacon, cooked crisp and crumbled

1 large tomato, chopped

1/2 avocado, diced

Preheat oven to 325 degrees.

Heat a skillet over medium heat. Add 1/2 tablespoon oil and the onions and cook 4 minutes, until onions are soft. Stir in milk, flour, salt, and pepper. Cook until slightly thickened. Add cheese and stir until melted.

Layer the potatoes and cheese mixture in a 3-quart rectangular baking dish. Bake, covered, for 55 minutes, or until potatoes are tender.

Heat the remaining oil over medium heat. Add broccoli and cook until tender.

In a large bowl, beat the eggs and egg whites with 2 tablespoons water. Season with salt and pepper. Pour the egg mixture over the broccoli. Cook, stirring, over medium heat until eggs are set. Spoon egg mixture over the potatoes and top with crumbled bacon, tomatoes, and avocado.

NUTRITION PER SERVING | FAT: 15 GRAMS | CARBOHYDRATE: 36 GRAMS | PROTEIN: 18 GRAMS | TOTAL CALORIES: 351

SUNRISE EGG MUFFIN

In much less time than it would take you to get in your car and go pick up breakfast at the drive-through window, you can whip up this delicious meal right in your own kitchen—plus get more nutrients than you would otherwise obtain from the fast-food alternative. The fast fuel here is the English muffin.

1 SERVING

1 large egg
1 slice Canadian bacon
1 whole-wheat English muffin, toasted

1 slice tomato
3 thin slices avocado

Coat a skillet with cooking spray and heat over medium-high heat. Crack the egg into the skillet and cook for 1–2 minutes on each side, depending on how you like your eggs cooked. Remove the egg and set aside.

Using the same skillet, cook the Canadian bacon for 1 minute on each side. Place the bottom of the muffin on a plate and top with the egg. Add Canadian bacon, tomato, and avocado and top with the other half of the muffin.

NUTRITION PER SERVING FAT: 13 GRAMS CARBOHYDRATE: 31 GRAMS PROTEIN: 25 GRAMS TOTAL CALORIES: 341

BROCCOLI AND GOAT CHEESE OMELET WITH TOAST

The secret ingredient here is goat cheese—it melts beautifully and tastes distinctively delicious. Goat cheese is easier on the digestive system (that's a plus for me, since I'm a tad lactose-intolerant) and is lower in calories than cheese made from cow's milk. The toast supplies some fast fuel.

1 SERVING

1 cup chopped broccoli

2 large eggs, beaten

1/2 teaspoon chopped fresh dill, or 1/4 teaspoon dried

1 scallion, chopped

2 tablespoons crumbled goat cheese

2 slices whole-wheat bread, toasted

Coat a skillet with cooking spray and heat over medium heat. Add broccoli and cook until tender.

Combine eggs and dill. Pour egg mixture into the pan with the broccoli and cook 3 minutes, until set. Add scallion and cheese.

Fold the omelet in half and serve with toast.

NUTRITION PER SERVING | FAT: 16 GRAMS | CARBOHYDRATE: 39 GRAMS | PROTEIN: 24 GRAMS | TOTAL CALORIES: 396

HANGOVER BREAKFAST SANDWICH

After a night of celebrations—or of bad decisions!—we tend to crave grease and carbs. Here's a recipe that solves that craving but without all the bad fats and sugars. The mayo-lemon sauce approximates Hollandaise, so the whole thing feels a little decadent. It's not! (It's not just a hangover cure, either; this meal is great any day of the week.)

1 SERVING

2 tablespoons low-fat mayonnaise

1 teaspoon lemon juice

1/8 teaspoon cayenne

2 slices Canadian bacon

1 whole-wheat English muffin

1/2 cup tightly packed baby spinach

1 large egg

2 slices tomato

2 slices avocado

Preheat the oven to 400 degrees. Coat a baking sheet with cooking spray.

In a small bowl, whisk together the mayonnaise, lemon juice, and cayenne. Season with salt and pepper. Set aside.

Arrange the bacon slices and the two halves of the muffin separately on the baking sheet and bake for 10 minutes. Place the spinach on top of the bacon slices and bake 2–3 minutes more, until the spinach is wilted.

Coat a small skillet with cooking spray and heat over medium-high heat. Crack the egg into the skillet and season with salt and pepper. Cook until the egg white is opaque and edges are crispy.

On a plate, layer the bottom half of the English muffin with egg, half the bacon, and spinach, then with half the tomatoes and avocado. Drizzle with half the mayonnaise mixture. Layer with the remaining bacon and spinach, tomatoes, and avocado, and drizzle with the rest of the mayonnaise mixture. Top with the other half of the English muffin.

NUTRITION PER SERVING | **FAT: 14 GRAMS** | CARBOHYDRATE: 24 GRAMS | **PROTEIN: 14 GRAMS** | **TOTAL CALORIES: 278**

TROPICAL AÇAI BOWL

V

Here's a refreshing breakfast that makes use of açai (ah-SIGH-ee). Hailing from the Amazon rainforest, the açai berry is one of the richest fruit sources of antioxidants, possibly possessing age-defying and cancer-fighting benefits. In this recipe, I've used açai puree, which you can buy in convenient frozen packs.

1 SERVING

One 8-ounce pack unsweetened frozen açai puree
1 tablespoon agave syrup
1/2 cup blueberries

1 small banana, sliced
1/2 cup pineapple chunks
1 scoop plant-based protein powder
1 tablespoon granola

Combine the açai puree, agave, half the blueberries, half the banana, half the pineapple chunks, and the protein powder in a blender. Blend until thick and smooth.

Transfer to a bowl and top with the remaining fruit and the granola.

NUTRITION PER SERVING | FAT: 12 GRAMS | CARBOHYDRATE: 82 GRAMS | PROTEIN: 27 GRAMS | TOTAL CALORIES: 544

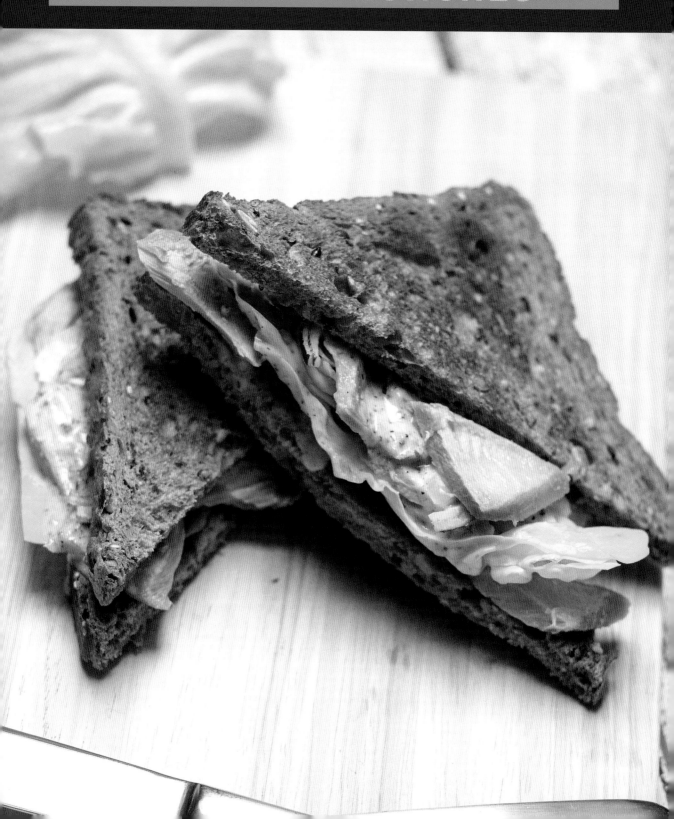

SALMON SALAD SANDWICH

Canned tuna was one of my favorite pantry staples until I read that some types of canned tuna may contain more mercury than previously thought. Even though I still enjoy a good tuna salad sandwich from time to time, I decided to turn my favorite tuna salad sandwich into one made with canned salmon, which apparently is still safe. *Voilà:* I'm happy to present this fantastic-tasting sandwich. The whole-grain bread is the fast fuel.

2 SERVINGS

One 4-ounce can salmon packed in water, drained

1/4 cup finely chopped celery

2 tablespoons finely chopped red onions

1 tablespoon low-fat mayonnaise

11/2 teaspoons brown mustard

11/2 teaspoons olive oil

11/2 teaspoons lemon juice

11/2 teaspoons pepper

1/2 teaspoon kosher salt (or coarse Himalayan salt, if you have it)

2 leaves butter lettuce

4 slices whole-grain bread

Combine all ingredients except lettuce and bread and mix well. Allow the salmon mixture to sit for about 30 minutes in the refrigerator before assembling it into a sandwich with the bread and lettuce.

NUTRITION PER SERVING FAT: 8 GRAMS CARBOHYDRATE: 39 GRAMS PROTEIN: 18 GRAMS TOTAL CALORIES: 300

SALMON SOBA NOODLE BOWL

If you've never heard of soba noodles, let me introduce you to this fast fuel. A staple in the Japanese diet, soba is a type of noodle made from buckwheat and wheat flour. It can be as fine as angel-hair pasta or as thick as fettuccine. Buckwheat has twice the energy-promoting B vitamins as wheat. Enjoy these healthful noodles in this delicious blend of salmon and veggies.

2 SERVINGS

4 ounces dried soba (buckwheat) noodles

5 ounces asparagus, cut into 1-inch pieces

4 ounces skinless salmon fillet, cut into
  8 pieces

1 tablespoon sesame oil

3 tablespoons lime juice

4 ounces cucumber, peeled and diced

2 ounces shredded carrots

1/2 small avocado, diced

Cook the noodles in boiling water for 6 minutes. With tongs, transfer the noodles to a strainer and drain. Add asparagus to the same boiling water and cook 2 minutes; rinse under cold water.

Coat a skillet with cooking spray and heat over medium-high heat. Cook salmon for 2–3 minutes on each side, until cooked through. Set aside.

In a bowl, whisk together the oil and lime juice; season with salt and pepper. Add the noodles, asparagus, cucumber, carrots, and avocado and toss lightly.

NUTRITION PER SERVING | FAT: 16 GRAMS | CARBOHYDRATE: 47 GRAMS | PROTEIN: 24 GRAMS | TOTAL CALORIES: 428

CHICKEN COLESLAW SALAD

Chicken breasts are the fallback meal when we diet, and for good reason: chicken is low in fat, inexpensive, and high in protein. But it comes with a price—boredom. The trick is changing up the way you prepare your chicken breasts. Here's a salad that will help you do just that. The addition of the apple turns this dish into a fast-fuel meal.

4 SERVINGS

1 tablespoon olive oil
2 skinless, boneless chicken breasts
2 tablespoons pumpkin seeds
2 tablespoons sunflower seeds
1 cup plain low-fat yogurt
1 teaspoon white vinegar
1 teaspoon apple cider vinegar

1 teaspoon lemon juice
1 tablespoon sugar
2 cups shredded red cabbage
1 cup shredded kale
1 large apple, cored and cut into small cubes
2 celery stalks, cut into thin strips
1 large carrot, shredded

Heat a skillet over medium-high heat. Add oil and cook chicken for about 10–12 minutes on each side, until done. Remove and cut into small pieces.

Heat another skillet over medium heat. Toast the pumpkin and sunflower seeds 3–4 minutes, stirring often, until the seeds are fragrant and beginning to color.

In a small bowl, whisk together the yogurt, vinegars, lemon juice, and sugar. Season with salt and pepper.

Place the chicken, cabbage, kale, apple, celery, and carrots in a large bowl and toss gently. Add yogurt dressing and toss with pumpkin and sunflower seeds.

NUTRITION PER SERVING | FAT: 11 GRAMS | CARBOHYDRATE: 19 GRAMS | PROTEIN: 18 GRAMS | TOTAL CALORIES: 247

CHICKEN ORZO SALAD

Orzo is a small, rice-shaped pasta that is classified as a fast fuel. As with any type of pasta, it makes a great salad addition, especially when mixed with a power protein such as chicken breast. This recipe makes 4 servings, so feel free to store extra servings for later.

4 SERVINGS

¾ cup whole-wheat orzo

1 tablespoon olive oil

3 tablespoons lemon juice

½ teaspoon minced garlic

¼ teaspoon agave syrup

1 cup shredded skinless, boneless rotisserie chicken breast

½ cup diced English cucumber

½ cup chopped red bell peppers

⅓ cup thinly sliced scallions

1 cup tightly packed baby arugula

2 tablespoons chopped fresh dill

½ cup crumbled goat cheese

Cook orzo according to package directions. Drain and set aside.

In a large bowl, whisk together the oil, lemon juice, garlic, and agave. Add the chicken, vegetables, dill, and drained orzo. Season with salt and pepper and toss well. Top with goat cheese.

NUTRITION PER SERVING FAT: 9 GRAMS CARBOHYDRATE: 15 GRAMS PROTEIN: 19 GRAMS TOTAL CALORIES: 217

HOO-YA

SALTS OF THE EARTH

Did you know that salt is the only rock we eat? That's right. It's an important element in our diets (as long as we don't overdo it). Salt contains minerals vital to health, and it enhances the flavor of many foods, helping us to eat a varied diet. Plus, it has served as an effective way to preserve meat, fish, and vegetables.

These days, you can choose from many different types of salt. In my cooking, I use regular table salt, the most common refined salt. It does contain additives, including anti-caking agents, so that it flows freely from the shaker. Most table salts contain iodine, needed for health and metabolism.

There are two specialty salts I like for recipes. The first is kosher salt, a coarse-grained salt that does not contain iodine, imparting a fresher, cleaner taste. Many chefs and gourmet cooks prefer to cook with kosher salt because of its texture and flavor. The other salt I like is pink Himalayan salt, which is mined from ancient sea salt deposits in the Himalayas and contains eighty-four minerals, including iron.

If you choose to cook with salt or salt your foods, go easy. Too much salt in the diet can lead to high blood pressure. Nutrition experts caution against eating more than 1 teaspoon of salt daily.

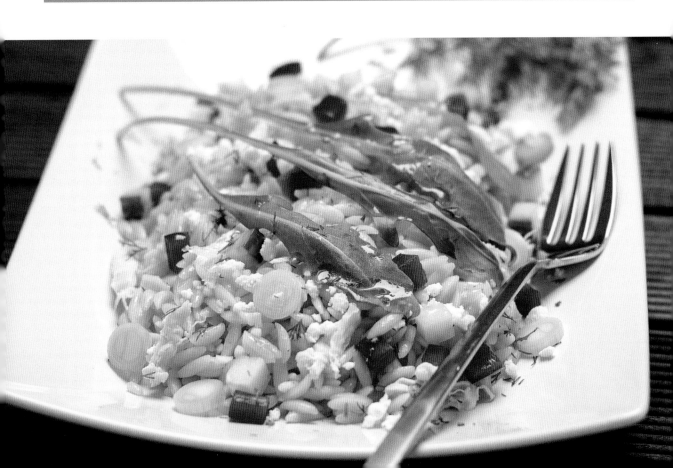

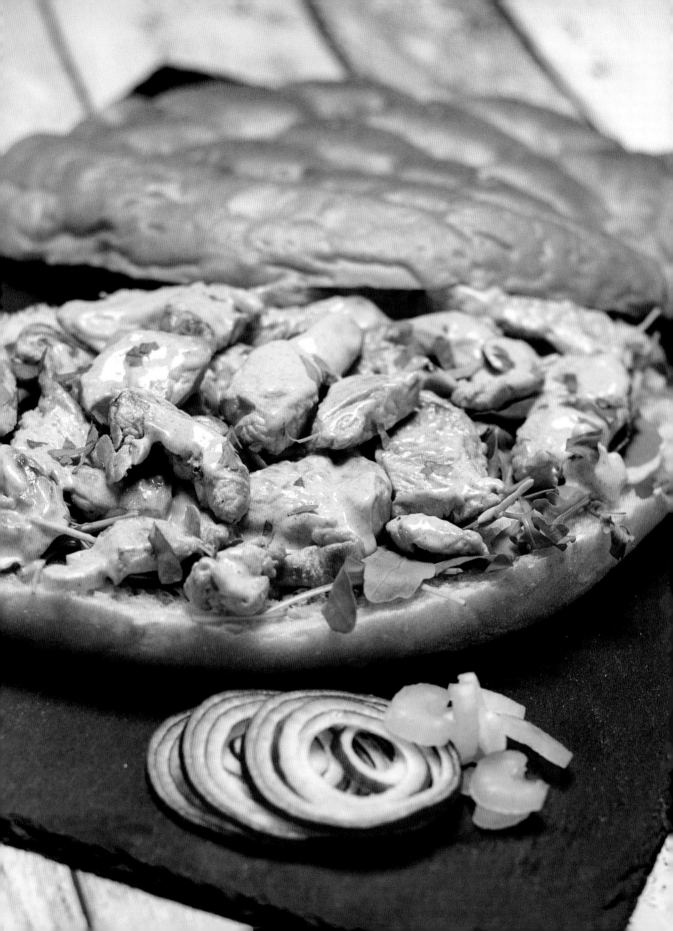

CHICKEN CURRY WRAPS

Curry has been touted for its ability to fight cancer, viruses, inflammation, and more. What I like best about curry, though, is its ability to spice up meals, from stews to yummy chicken wraps like these. The whole-grain wraps are fast fuels.

2 SERVINGS

1 cup shredded skinless, boneless rotisserie chicken breast

1/4 teaspoon kosher salt (or coarse Himalayan salt, if you have it)

1/2 cup plain low-fat yogurt

1 garlic clove, minced

11/2 teaspoons lime juice

1/4 cup sliced celery

11/2 tablespoons curry powder

2 whole-grain wraps or 1 baguette sliced in half

1 cup tightly packed baby arugula

1/8 red onion, thinly sliced

1/4 bunch cilantro, chopped

In a bowl, toss together the chicken, salt, yogurt, garlic, lime juice, celery, and curry powder. Cover and marinate in the refrigerator at least 21/2 hours.

Spread the chicken mixture over the wraps or baguette slices and top with arugula, onions, and cilantro. If making wraps, roll up both wraps tightly.

NUTRITION PER SERVING | FAT: 9 GRAMS | CARBOHYDRATE: 32 GRAMS | PROTEIN: 42 GRAMS | TOTAL CALORIES: 377

HAWAIIAN BBQ CHICKEN PIZZA

An entire 12-inch deep-dish Hawaiian pizza could deliver more than 3,500 calories, or more than 650 calories a slice. That's a fat-gaining disaster, for sure. Here's a delicious version that cuts those calories in half and boosts the nutrition considerably, thanks to a fast fuel in the form of whole-wheat tortillas and barbecue sauce.

4 SERVINGS

1 cup shredded skinless, boneless rotisserie chicken breast

1/2 cup barbecue sauce

4 whole-wheat tortillas

1/2 tablespoon olive oil

1/2 small red onion, thinly sliced

1/2 cup pineapple chunks

3 ounces shredded reduced-fat mozzarella

1/2 cup chopped cilantro

Preheat oven to 425 degrees. Coat a baking sheet with cooking spray. In a small bowl, toss chicken and sauce.

Place tortillas on the baking sheet and brush with oil. Divide the chicken, onions, and pineapple chunks between them. Sprinkle with mozzarella.

Bake until the cheese is melted and the bottoms of the tortillas are lightly brown, 5–7 minutes. Sprinkle with cilantro and slice into wedges.

NUTRITION PER SERVING	FAT: 8 GRAMS	CARBOHYDRATE: 49 GRAMS	PROTEIN: 28 GRAMS	TOTAL CALORIES: 372

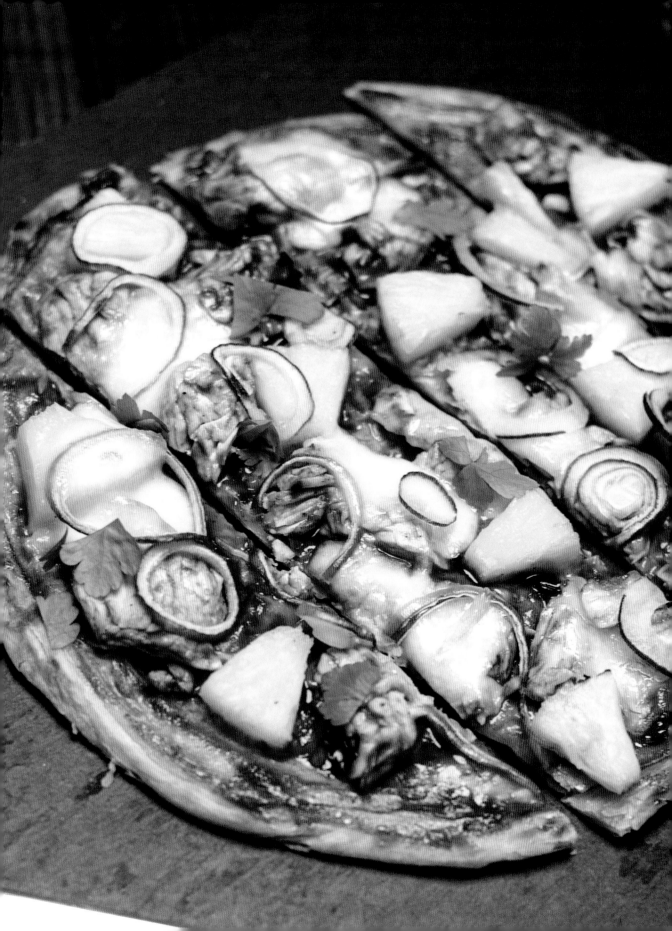

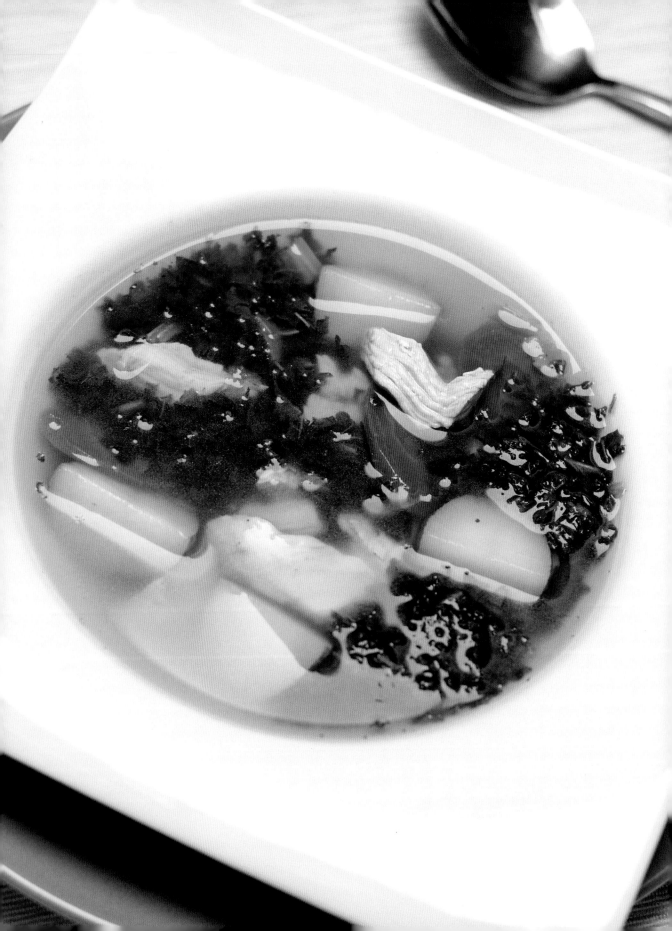

CHICKEN KALE SOUP

I love a steaming pot of chicken soup. Hey, it's a cure for everything, right? For a slight twist, I've added the super-green kale to it, so now this traditional soup is not only more healthful but also more colorful. The fast-fuel potatoes supply extra carbohydrates for energy.

4 SERVINGS

2 skinless, boneless chicken breasts

10 black peppercorns

Four 14.5-ounce cans low-sodium, low-fat chicken broth

6 small Yukon Gold potatoes, quartered

1 cup chopped carrots

1/2 pound kale, chopped

1 cup chopped celery

1 teaspoon black pepper

1 tablespoon kosher salt (or coarse Himalayan salt, if you have it)

Place chicken and peppercorns in a large pot, cover with water, and bring to a boil. Simmer 20 minutes, until chicken is cooked through. Remove chicken from pot, cool, and shred the meat.

In another large pot, combine the chicken broth, potatoes, carrots, kale, celery, pepper, and salt. Bring to a boil, then reduce heat and simmer 30 minutes. Add chicken and cook for another 10 minutes. Adjust seasonings.

NUTRITION PER SERVING | FAT: 4 GRAMS | CARBOHYDRATE: 36 GRAMS | PROTEIN: 33 GRAMS | TOTAL CALORIES: 312

CHICKEN AND WHITE BEAN SOUP

Nothing warms body and soul like a bowl of soothing, satisfying soup, and it doesn't hurt that most soups are quick and inexpensive to make. This one freezes well, so make a large batch in order to have leftovers another day. Just place your cooled soup in airtight, freezer-safe containers, leaving about a half-inch of room at the top to allow for expansion during freezing.

4 SERVINGS

1 tablespoon olive oil

6 garlic cloves, minced

1 cup chopped onions

4 cups chopped spinach

4 cups low-sodium, low-fat chicken broth

1 cup shredded skinless, boneless rotisserie chicken breast

1/2 cup chopped carrots

1 large tomato, chopped

Two 15-ounce cans cannellini beans, drained and rinsed

1 tablespoon chopped fresh thyme

1 tablespoon chopped fresh rosemary

1 teaspoon black pepper

1 tablespoon Himalayan salt

1/2 cup chopped fresh chives

Heat a large pot over medium-high heat. Add oil, garlic, and onions and cook 2–3 minutes, until the onions have softened. Add spinach and cook 1–2 minutes, until wilted. Add 3 cups broth, the chicken, carrots, tomatoes, 2 cups beans, the thyme, rosemary, pepper, and salt and simmer 10 minutes. Place the remaining broth and beans in a blender and blend until smooth. Add the bean puree to the soup and simmer 15–20 minutes more. Garnish with chives.

NUTRITION PER SERVING | FAT: 12 GRAMS | CARBOHYDRATE: 42 GRAMS | PROTEIN: 29 GRAMS | TOTAL CALORIES: 392

MEDITERRANEAN CHICKEN WRAPS

Research shows that folks who eat a Mediterranean diet are often the healthiest people on earth, with lower rates of heart disease, stroke, and cancer than people who eat less healthfully. Here's a great way to get all the goodness of Mediterranean food in a single fast-fuel wrap.

3 SERVINGS

1/2 cup shredded skinless, boneless rotisserie chicken breast

1 small cucumber, chopped

1/2 tablespoon olive oil

1/2 cup grape tomatoes, halved

11/2 tablespoons chopped pitted Kalamata olives

1/2 tablespoon chopped onions

3/4 tablespoon lemon juice

1 tablespoon crumbled feta cheese

1/2 tablespoon chopped fresh oregano

Pinch cayenne

Three 8-inch whole-wheat tortillas

3 tablespoons plain hummus

Combine all ingredients except the tortillas and hummus in a bowl and mix well. Spread 1 tablespoon hummus on one side of each of the tortillas. Divide the chicken mixture among the tortillas, roll up, and cut in half.

| NUTRITION PER SERVING | FAT: 10 GRAMS | CARBOHYDRATE: 29 GRAMS | PROTEIN: 17 GRAMS | TOTAL CALORIES: 274 |

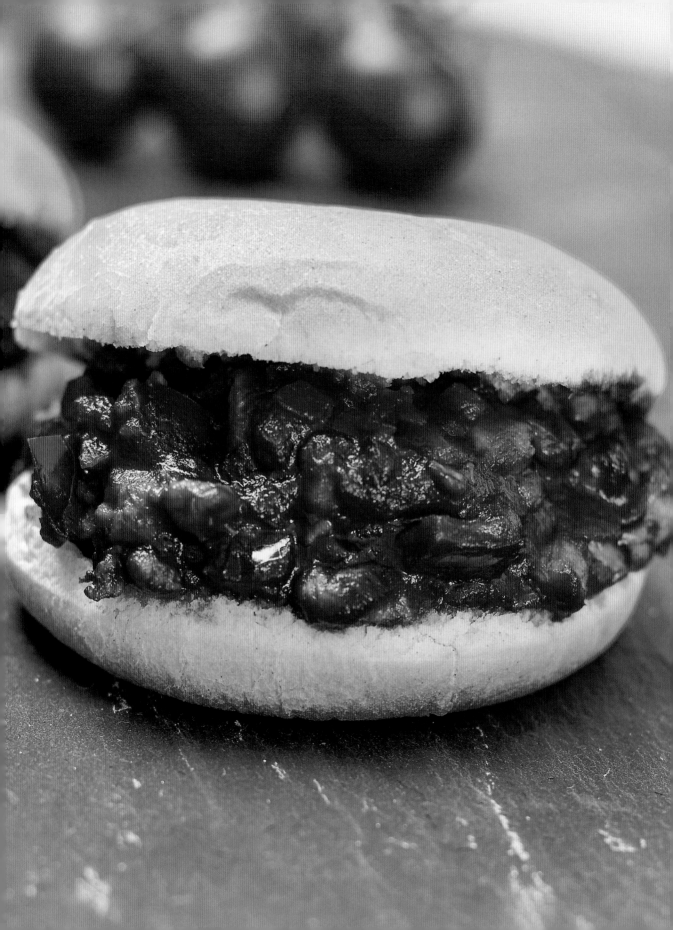

GUILT-FREE SLOPPY JOE

The sloppy Joe was invented during the Depression, when cash-strapped families stretched meat recipes by adding various tasty fillers. Traditionally, the dish has been made of ground beef and ketchup cooked in a skillet. I've toned down the calories and fat in my version. Served between fast-fuel buns, these sloppy Joes are filling and delicious.

6 SERVINGS

1 tablespoon olive oil

11/2 pounds ground turkey

1 tablespoon brown sugar

1 medium onion, diced

5 garlic cloves, minced

1 teaspoon dry mustard

1 large red bell pepper, diced

1 tablespoon red wine vinegar

11/2 tablespoons Worcestershire sauce

2 teaspoons chili powder

2 cups tomato sauce

2 tablespoons tomato paste

6 hamburger buns, toasted

Heat olive oil in a large skillet over medium heat. Brown the ground turkey, breaking up the meat as it cooks. Add the sugar, onion, garlic, mustard, and bell peppers and cook 3–5 minutes, until the vegetables have softened. Season with salt and pepper.

Add vinegar, Worcestershire sauce, chili powder, tomato sauce, and tomato paste and stir. Reduce heat to low and simmer, uncovered, 15 minutes, stirring often. Spoon the filling onto the buns.

NUTRITION PER SERVING | FAT: 13 GRAMS | CARBOHYDRATE: 34 GRAMS | PROTEIN: 25 GRAMS | TOTAL CALORIES: 353

TEX-MEX CORN AND AVOCADO SALAD

Tex-Mex is a fusion of Mexican and southwestern American cuisines. It's characterized by its heavy use of cheese, beef and pork, beans, and spices. In this recipe, I've spared the cheese and replaced it with avocado, which has healthful fats (and is also often found in Tex-Mex cuisine). Turkey bacon gives the salad a delicious meaty kick. There's a lot of fat-fighting fiber, too, in every bite, thanks to three fast fuels: black beans, corn, and tangerines.

2 SERVINGS

3 slices turkey bacon

11/2 tablespoons lime juice

1/2 tablespoon apple cider vinegar

1/2 tablespoon agave syrup

1/2 tablespoon olive oil

6 cherry tomatoes, quartered

1/4 cup finely chopped red onions

1/4 cup chopped red bell peppers

1 cup shredded kale

Half a 15-ounce can black beans, drained and rinsed

1/2 cup corn kernels

1/2 cup coarsely chopped cilantro

1 small tangerine, peeled, sectioned, and chopped

1/2 large avocado, cut into cubes

Cook turkey bacon until crisp and drain on paper towels; set aside.

In a small bowl, whisk the lime juice, vinegar, agave syrup, and oil. Season with salt and pepper.

In a large bowl, toss the tomatoes, onions, bell peppers, kale, beans, corn, cilantro, and tangerine. Crumble the bacon over the top, drizzle with the dressing, and toss gently. Top with avocado.

NUTRITION PER SERVING | FAT: 16 GRAMS | CARBOHYDRATE: 40 GRAMS | PROTEIN: 11 GRAMS | TOTAL CALORIES: 348

CHICKEN WITH STRAWBERRIES AND SPINACH SALAD

There's a lot you can do with strawberries besides dipping them in chocolate or eating them on shortcake. A fast fuel, strawberries make a perfect addition to a spinach salad, made all the sweeter with another fast fuel—figs—tossed in. The dressing is a flavorful combo of white wine vinegar, brown sugar, and fragrant basil. The crowning touch is the goat cheese and toasted almonds sprinkled on at serving time.

4 SERVINGS

2 skinless, boneless chicken breasts, cubed

2 tablespoons white wine vinegar

1 tablespoon olive oil

1 teaspoon brown sugar

2 tablespoons chopped fresh basil

1/4 red onion, thinly sliced

2 16-ounce bags baby spinach

1 cup strawberries, halved

1/4 cup dried figs, sliced

1/4 cup chopped toasted almonds

1/2 cup crumbled goat cheese

Coat a skillet with cooking spray and heat over medium-high heat. Sauté chicken until cooked through and lightly browned. Set aside to cool.

In a small bowl, whisk together the vinegar, oil, sugar, and basil. Set aside.

In a large bowl, combine the chicken, onions, spinach, strawberries, and figs and toss gently. Drizzle with dressing and top with the almonds and cheese. Season with salt and pepper.

NUTRITION PER SERVING | FAT: 13 GRAMS | CARBOHYDRATE: 18 GRAMS | PROTEIN: 21 GRAMS | TOTAL CALORIES: 273

SOUTHWESTERN ORZO SALAD

Here's another great-tasting Tex-Mex salad with an Italian touch, thanks to the addition of orzo, a fast fuel. I love all foods and all cuisines so much that I see no problem in trying to fuse several in one dish, as this salad does.

6 SERVINGS

1 cup whole-wheat orzo

1 cup canned whole-kernel corn

1/2 cup canned black beans, rinsed and drained

One 12-ounce can chicken breast in water, drained and shredded

12 cherry tomatoes, quartered

3 scallions, chopped

3 tablespoons chopped cilantro

1/4 cup olive oil

3 tablespoons lime juice

1 teaspoon chili powder

1/2 teaspoon kosher salt

1/2 teaspoon black pepper

1/4 teaspoon crushed red pepper

1 avocado, sliced

Cook orzo according to package directions. Drain, rinse with cold water, and drain thoroughly. In a large bowl, toss orzo, corn, beans, chicken, tomatoes, scallions, and cilantro.

In a small bowl, whisk oil, lime juice, chili powder, salt, pepper, and crushed red pepper. Toss salad with the dressing and top with avocado.

NUTRITION PER SERVING | FAT: 15 GRAMS | CARBOHYDRATE: 26 GRAMS | PROTEIN: 17 GRAMS | TOTAL CALORIES: 307

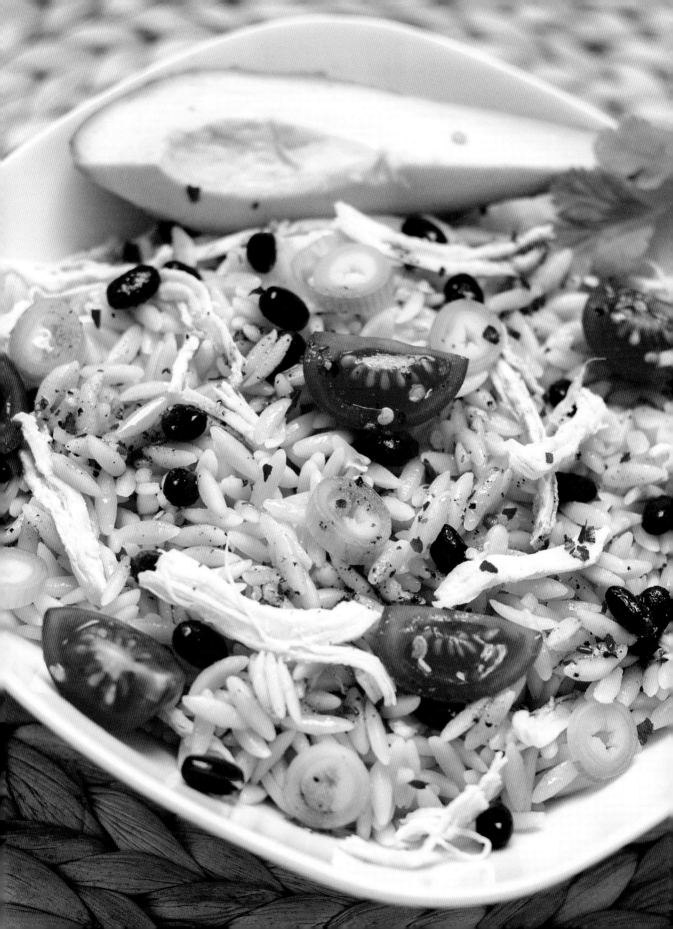

PESTO STEAK SANDWICH

To my mind (and mouth), nothing beats pesto as a sandwich spread, especially mixed with a little mayo to thin it out. Pesto is a classic Italian sauce usually made from a heavenly blend of basil, olive oil, pine nuts, garlic, and cheese. The basil is not only tasty but also an excellent source of vitamin K and a very good source of iron. Spread it on crusty bread and top with the ingredients below, and you've got a hearty, healthful sandwich.

2 SERVINGS

8-ounce London broil, trimmed
1/4 teaspoon Montreal steak seasoning
1/8 teaspoon salt
1/8 teaspoon pepper
1/4 teaspoon garlic powder
1 tablespoon store-bought pesto

1 tablespoon low-fat mayonnaise
2 ciabatta rolls, toasted
1/2 cup tightly packed baby arugula
1 tomato, sliced
1/8 red onion, thinly sliced

Trim excess fat from the steak. Combine the Montreal steak seasoning, salt, pepper, and garlic powder in a small bowl. Rub the steak with the spice mixture and let sit at room temperature for an hour.

Preheat the grill to medium heat. Grill steak 3 to 5 minutes on each side, until done to your liking. Transfer to a plate and let rest 5 minutes.

Combine pesto and mayo in a small bowl and mix well.

Cut the ciabatta rolls in half and spread the pesto mixture evenly over each side of the bread. Layer bottom of each piece of bread with steak, arugula, tomatoes, and onions, and top with the other half of the bread.

NUTRITION PER SERVING | FAT: 14 GRAMS | CARBOHYDRATE: 33 GRAMS | PROTEIN: 32 GRAMS | TOTAL CALORIES: 386

CREAM OF WHEAT SOUP (GRIESS KNOEDEL SUPPE)

I live in Germany much of every year and have come to love the luncheon tradition of dumpling soup served with liverwurst sandwiches. What I could do without, however, is all the fat that comes from the frying of the dumplings in traditional recipes. In my much less fattening version, the dumplings cook in boiling broth, soaking up the brothy flavor with no frying required.

3 SERVINGS

1 chicken bouillon cube
1/2 teaspoon salt
Pinch ground nutmeg
1/2 tablespoon butter
1/2 cup cream of wheat
1 large egg, beaten
1 scallion, chopped

SANDWICH
3 slices rye bread
Mustard (optional)
3 tablespoons liverwurst spread
Sliced onions (optional)
Dill pickle slices (optional)

Combine chicken bouillon cube with 4 cups water and bring to a boil over medium-high heat. Reduce heat and keep at a simmer.

In another pot, bring 1 cup plus 2 tablespoons water, the salt, nutmeg, and butter to a boil. Add cream of wheat, turn heat to low, and cook, stirring, until the cream of wheat has a thick, doughy consistency. Remove pot from heat and stir in the egg.

Drop the cream of wheat mixture by spoonfuls into the simmering broth. The dumplings are done when they float to the top. Add scallion.

Spread each piece of rye bread with mustard if desired. Add liverwurst. Top with onions and pickles if using. Serve with soup.

NUTRITION PER SERVING | FAT: 8 GRAMS | CARBOHYDRATE: 44 GRAMS | PROTEIN: 12 GRAMS | TOTAL CALORIES: 296

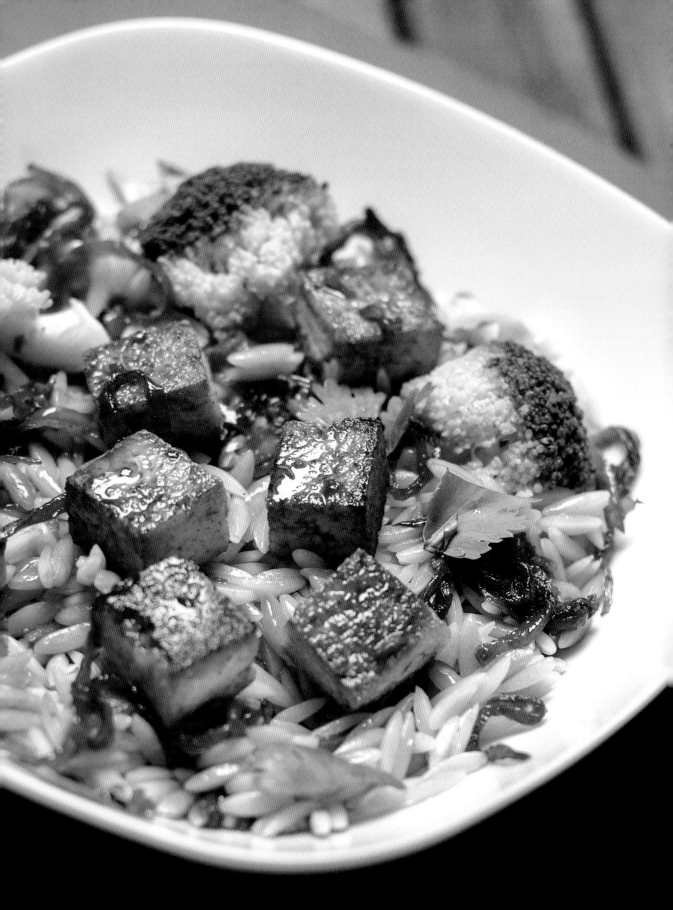

TOFU ORZO BOWL

V

Every so often, I go meatless and turn to tofu as a protein substitute for meat. No matter what you think of tofu, understand that it doesn't have much of a taste by itself; it takes on the flavors of whatever it's combined with. This pasta dish, for example, has a great Asian flavor, thanks to the sauces used. Tofu pairs beautifully with the fast-fuel orzo, too.

1 SERVING

1/3 cup whole-wheat orzo

1 teaspoon olive oil

1/4 cup chopped onions

1 garlic clove, minced

4 ounces firm tofu, cubed

11/2 cups frozen stir-fry vegetables

1 tablespoon Mrs. Dash Spicy Teriyaki Marinade or any teriyaki sauce

1/2 tablespoon low-sodium soy sauce

Sriracha (optional)

Chopped cilantro

Cook orzo according to the package directions. Drain the orzo, reserving 1/2 cup cooking water.

In a skillet, heat olive oil over medium-high heat and cook the onions, garlic, and tofu for 2 minutes. Add vegetables, 1 tablespoon reserved cooking water, teriyaki marinade, and soy sauce and cook for 2 minutes more.

Stir in the orzo. Add more reserved cooking water if needed.

Add sriracha if desired. Garnish with cilantro.

NUTRITION PER SERVING | FAT: 14 GRAMS | CARBOHYDRATE: 32 GRAMS | PROTEIN: 16 GRAMS | TOTAL CALORIES: 318

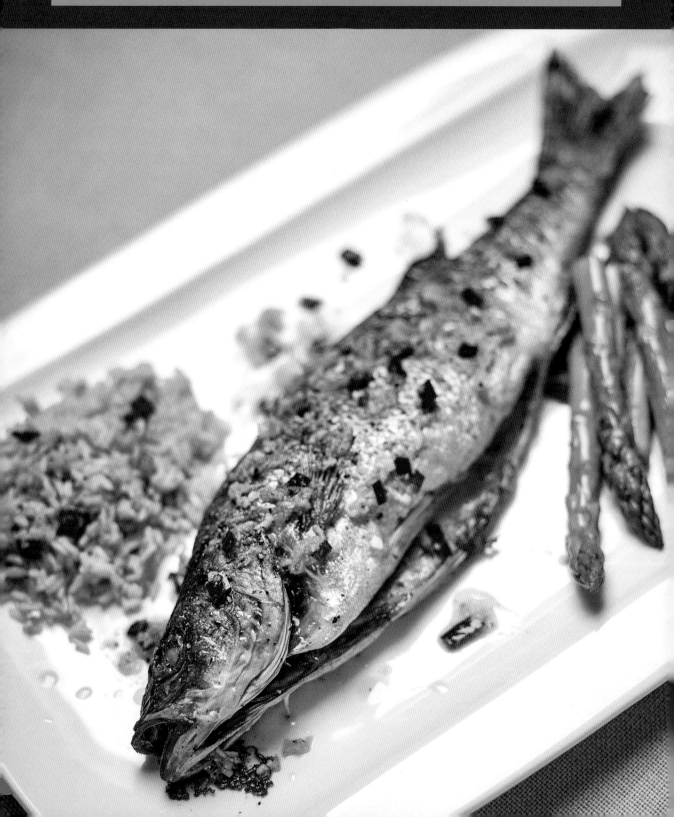

FAST-FUEL DINNERS

GINGER SEA BASS

Sea bass is a mild white fish and works well with any number of spices and marinades. In this recipe, the ginger balances out the spiciness of the chile and garlic and adds a delicious twist. The brown rice makes it a satisfying fast-fuel dinner.

4 SERVINGS

2 cups brown rice

Four 6-ounce wild sea bass fillets (or two whole fish)

3 tablespoons fish sauce

2 tablespoons grated ginger

1 tablespoon brown sugar

2 garlic cloves, minced

1 red or green chile, minced

2 tablespoons lime juice

1 tablespoon olive oil

1 bunch asparagus, ends trimmed and stalks cut in half

Preheat oven to 375 degrees.

Cook the rice according to package directions and set aside.

Coat a baking sheet with cooking spray. Place sea bass on the sheet, season with salt and pepper, and bake 20–30 minutes, until slightly golden.

In a small bowl, whisk together the fish sauce, ginger, 1/4 cup water, sugar, half the garlic, the chiles, and lime juice.

Preheat a large skillet or wok over medium-high heat. Add olive oil and the remaining garlic and cook 1–2 minutes, until garlic is lightly golden. Add asparagus and stir-fry 5–7 minutes, until tender.

Transfer sea bass to plates, drizzle with ginger-garlic sauce, and serve with asparagus and rice.

NUTRITION PER SERVING | FAT: 10 GRAMS | CARBOHYDRATE: 30 GRAMS | PROTEIN: 53 GRAMS | TOTAL CALORIES: 422

CORIANDER BAKED SALMON

Here's a fish recipe sizzling with flavor, thanks to its crust of coriander seeds. You might be more familiar with coriander in its leaf form cilantro. Coriander is used medicinally as well as in various international cuisines. You'll love what it does for salmon, which teams up with wild rice, a fast fuel.

3 SERVINGS

1 tablespoon coriander seeds, crushed
11/2 teaspoons salt
11/2 teaspoons black pepper
1 tablespoon olive oil
Three 3-ounce salmon fillets

1 cup wild rice
1 cup fresh green beans
2 garlic cloves, minced
1/2 lemon, cut into wedges

Preheat oven to 375 degrees.

Combine the crushed coriander, salt, pepper, and 1/2 tablespoon oil. Coat salmon with this mixture. Allow to sit for 15–30 minutes.

Cook rice according to package directions and set aside.

Place the salmon on a baking sheet and bake 20–30 minutes, until the fish flakes easily with a fork.

Heat a skillet over high heat. Add the remaining oil, green beans, and garlic. Stir-fry 5–7 minutes, until green beans are tender. Season with salt and pepper. Divide the salmon, green beans, and wild rice among three plates and serve with lemon wedges.

NUTRITION PER SERVING | FAT: 10 GRAMS | CARBOHYDRATE: 20 GRAMS | PROTEIN: 35 GRAMS | TOTAL CALORIES: 320

SPICY SHRIMP AND WILD RICE

This recipe is perfect for entertaining. It doesn't take long to make, and your guests won't even know that it's healthful and lean. The spices give it a Cajun flavor that complements the shrimp without being too fiery. The wild rice in this recipe is a fast fuel.

4 SERVINGS

1 pound large shrimp, peeled and deveined

3 garlic cloves, minced

1 tablespoon Creole seasoning

1 teaspoon cayenne

1/4 cup lemon juice

4 sprigs leaves from fresh thyme

2 cups wild rice

1 teaspoon Himalayan salt

2 tablespoons olive oil

1 red bell pepper, chopped

1/4 cup chopped parsley

In a large bowl, toss the shrimp with the garlic, Creole seasoning, cayenne, lemon juice, and thyme. Marinate 20 minutes.

Cook wild rice according to package directions and set aside.

Heat a pan over medium-high heat, add oil and shrimp, and stir-fry until the shrimp begin to turn pink. Add the bell peppers and cook 2 minutes more, until the shrimp are cooked through. Add the parsley and season with Himalayan salt and pepper. Serve over the wild rice.

NUTRITION PER SERVING | FAT: 9 GRAMS | CARBOHYDRATE: 23 GRAMS | PROTEIN: 19 GRAMS | TOTAL CALORIES: 249

SESAME SEARED AHI TUNA

Here's a dish often served in upscale restaurants as either an appetizer or entrée. Now you can prepare it at home, and my version rivals what you'd order at the restaurant. Plus, cooking this delectable meal at home puts you in control of the ingredients—no worries about hidden fats, too much sugar, or other waistline-unfriendly additives. The addition of fast-fuel brown rice is the perfect complement. You can purchase ponzu (Japanese citrus-based sauce) through online suppliers, in the Asian aisle of your grocery store, or at Asian markets.

4 SERVINGS

1 cup brown rice

Four 6-ounce wild-caught ahi tuna fillets

2 tablespoons finely chopped ginger

2 tablespoons low-sodium soy sauce

1 tablespoon dry mustard

1 tablespoon honey

1 tablespoon olive oil

4 tablespoons sesame seeds

1/2 cup ponzu (Japanese citrus-based sauce)

3 tablespoons wasabi

Cook rice according to package directions and set aside.

Place the tuna in a large bowl. In a small bowl, whisk together ginger, soy sauce, mustard, honey, and oil. Pour ginger mixture over tuna and turn to coat. Sprinkle the fillets with sesame seeds.

Preheat grill to medium-high heat. Grill tuna 2 minutes on each side, until done to your liking. Serve with the rice. Pass ponzu and wasabi for dipping.

NUTRITION PER SERVING | FAT: 10 GRAMS | CARBOHYDRATE: 41 GRAMS | PROTEIN: 40 GRAMS | TOTAL CALORIES: 414

EDAMAME SPAGHETTI AND SHRIMP

Spaghetti has been widely reinvented—now you can find whole-wheat and gluten-free varieties, among others. One of the newest is edamame spaghetti. Because it's made with soybeans, it's super-high in protein and fiber, which makes it a great fast fuel.

2 SERVINGS

4 ounces edamame spaghetti

2 tablespoons olive oil

2 garlic cloves, minced

1/4 cup diced onions

12 large shrimp, peeled and deveined

1 cup tightly packed spinach

1 tablespoon lemon juice (optional)

1/2 cup chopped parsley

Cook spaghetti according to package directions; drain and set aside.

Heat a skillet over medium-high heat. Add oil, garlic, and onions and cook 2 minutes. Add shrimp and cook 2 minutes more, until shrimp are beginning to turn pink. Add spinach and cook for 1 minute more. Transfer to a big bowl.

Add noodles and lemon juice (if using) to shrimp, season with salt and pepper, and toss lightly. Top with parsley.

NUTRITION PER SERVING | FAT: 17 GRAMS | CARBOHYDRATE: 26 GRAMS | PROTEIN: 40 GRAMS | TOTAL CALORIES: 417

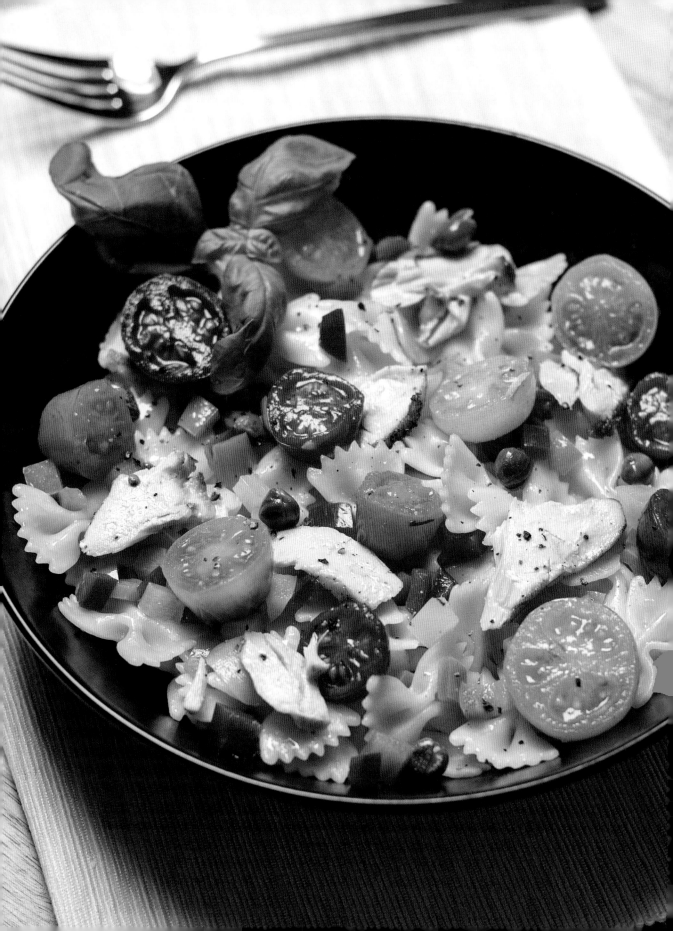

SALMON PASTA

Here's a fast-fuel dinner that looks too pretty to eat, with the bow-tie pasta and the vivid colors of the vegetables. But eat it I will! The more colorful a meal, the more vitamins and phytochemicals you're putting in your body. This is a healing dish that tastes good, too. Got leftovers? Refrigerate them, and serve this dish as a cold pasta salad tomorrow.

4 SERVINGS

16 ounces farfalle (bow-tie) pasta

16 ounces wild salmon

2 tablespoons olive oil

1 pound mixed sweet bell peppers, chopped

1 small package baby heirloom tomatoes, halved

2 tablespoons capers

1 tablespoon black pepper

3 garlic cloves, minced

2 sprigs fresh basil

Cook pasta as directed on package; drain and set aside.

Coat a skillet with cooking spray and heat over medium-high heat. Cook salmon for 5–7 minutes on each side, until cooked through. Set aside to cool.

In the same pan, combine oil, bell peppers, tomatoes, capers, black pepper, and garlic. Add pasta and stir-fry 5 minutes; season with salt. Place in a large serving dish. Break the salmon into large pieces and toss lightly with the pasta mixture. Garnish with basil.

NUTRITION PER SERVING | **FAT: 16 GRAMS** | **CARBOHYDRATE: 69 GRAMS** | **PROTEIN: 38 GRAMS** | **TOTAL CALORIES: 572**

CHICKEN CAPERS WITH ORZO

You've probably got the idea by now that I love orzo. If this fast-fuel were a celebrity, I'd be president of the fan club. Here orzo is paired with lean chicken cutlets and savory additions including capers, onions, and parsley.

4 SERVINGS

1 cup whole-wheat orzo

2 teaspoons grated lemon rind

Four 4-ounce chicken cutlets

1 tablespoon olive oil

1/4 cup white wine

1/2 cup diced onions

1/2 cup low-sodium, low-fat chicken broth

1 tablespoon lemon juice

1 tablespoon butter

2 tablespoons chopped parsley

1 tablespoon capers

Cook orzo according to the package directions. Drain; stir in lemon rind.

Season chicken with salt and pepper. Heat a large skillet over medium-high heat. Add oil and cook chicken 3 minutes on each side, until no longer pink in the middle. Remove chicken from the pan. Add wine and onions; cook 1 minute, scraping pan to loosen brown bits, until liquid has almost evaporated. Add broth and lemon juice; bring to a boil and cook for 2 minutes.

Remove from heat and add butter, parsley, and capers. Serve the chicken over the orzo and drizzle the pan sauce on top.

NUTRITION PER SERVING | FAT: 10 GRAMS | CARBOHYDRATE: 13 GRAMS | PROTEIN: 24 GRAMS | TOTAL CALORIES: 238

CHICKEN SCHNITZEL

Schnitzel is hugely popular in German cuisine, and traditionally it's made with pork. But I like to use chicken instead. I think it gives you the best of everything—lean protein, tasty herbs, and a consistency almost like chicken-fried steak. The bread crumbs are your fast fuel.

4 SERVINGS

2 cups tightly packed lettuce, or one 16-ounce bag of prewashed lettuce

1/2 cup cherry tomatoes

1/2 cucumber, thinly sliced

4 tablespoons olive oil

1/4 cup lemon juice

Four 6-ounce skinless, boneless chicken breasts

1 cup bread crumbs

1/2 cup grated low-fat Parmesan cheese

1/2 teaspoon dried thyme

1/2 teaspoon dried sage

1 large egg

2 garlic cloves, minced

1/2 teaspoon chopped parsley

4 lemon wedges

In a large bowl, combine lettuce, tomatoes, and the cucumber. In a small bowl, whisk 1 tablespoon oil, 1/2 cup water, and the lemon juice; season with salt and pepper. Set aside.

Place the chicken breasts between 2 sheets of heavy plastic wrap and pound to 1/2-inch thickness. Season both sides with salt and pepper.

In a shallow bowl, combine bread crumbs, cheese, thyme, and sage. In another shallow bowl, beat egg, garlic, and parsley; season with salt and pepper.

Dip each chicken breast in egg mixture, then in the bread crumb mixture, completely covering the chicken.

Heat a large skillet over medium-high heat. Add remaining 3 tablespoons oil and cook chicken 3 minutes on each side, until golden. Transfer to a plate; serve with lemon wedges. Add lemon dressing to salad and toss gently. Serve salad alongside chicken.

NUTRITION PER SERVING | FAT: 19 GRAMS | CARBOHYDRATE: 28 GRAMS | PROTEIN: 30 GRAMS | TOTAL CALORIES: 403

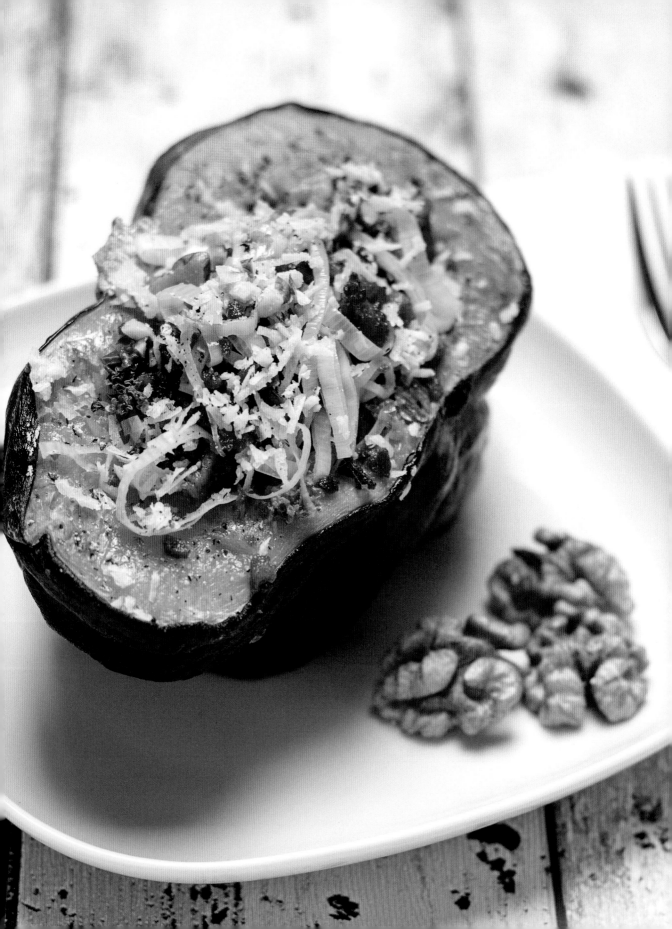

ACORN SQUASH WITH TURKEY SAUSAGE

I love acorn squash—not just because it's a fast fuel, high in fiber, and packed with vitamin A, but also because it tastes so good. Although acorn squash makes the perfect autumn meal, I can eat it at any time of the year. This recipe relies on high-protein turkey sausage as the stuffing base, making the dish a complete meal.

4 SERVINGS

2 acorn squash, halved, seeds removed

1/2 tablespoon olive oil

1/4 cup chopped onions

2 garlic cloves, minced

4 Italian turkey sausage links, casings removed

1 leek, white and light green parts only, sliced

4 cups tightly packed torn kale

1/3 cup low-sodium, low-fat chicken broth

2 tablespoons grated Parmesan cheese

2 tablespoons panko (Japanese-style bread crumbs)

1/4 cup chopped walnuts

Preheat oven to 375 degrees.

Coat squash with cooking spray and season with salt and pepper. Place cut side down on a baking sheet and bake 30 minutes, until soft. Remove from oven and set aside.

Heat a skillet over medium heat. Add olive oil and brown the onions and garlic. Crumble the sausage into the pan and cook 6 minutes, until brown. Add leeks, kale, and broth and cook 5 minutes more.

In a bowl, mix the Parmesan cheese, panko, and walnuts.

Divide sausage mixture among the squash halves and sprinkle the cheese mixture on top. Bake 2 minutes, until heated through.

NUTRITION PER SERVING | FAT: 12 GRAMS | CARBOHYDRATE: 31 GRAMS | PROTEIN: 27 GRAMS | TOTAL CALORIES: 340

SLOW COOKER CHICKEN AND RICE

One of my pet peeves is hearing the excuse "I don't have time to cook dinner." That's the same as saying you don't have time to invest in your health and well-being. Slow cooker to the rescue! It's the quickest and simplest way to cook dinner, and you can do it in a healthful way, as this recipe shows. The rice is your fast fuel.

4 SERVINGS

4 teaspoons salt

1 teaspoon cayenne

1 teaspoon thyme

2 teaspoons paprika

1 teaspoon onion powder

1 teaspoon white pepper

1/2 teaspoon black pepper

1/2 teaspoon garlic powder

1 whole roasting chicken

1 cup chopped onions

1 cup chopped carrots

1 cup brown rice

Combine the spices in a small bowl and set aside.

Remove any giblets from the cavity of the chicken, then rinse the chicken and pat dry. Rub spice mixture on chicken, place in plastic bag, and refrigerate overnight.

When ready to cook, put the onions and carrots at the bottom of the slow cooker. Add chicken and cook on low for 4–8 hours, until chicken is cooked through.

Cook rice according to package directions and serve with the chicken.

NUTRITION PER SERVING | FAT: 21 GRAMS | CARBOHYDRATE: 14 GRAMS | PROTEIN: 60 GRAMS | TOTAL CALORIES: 485

HOO-YA

SLOW COOKER TIPS

Slow cookers are the best time-savers for harried cooks, and just about any meal is suited for these handy cookers. Here are some tips I've found useful for making the most of them:

- Liquids don't evaporate from slow cookers, so you'll want to reduce the amount of liquid called for in a recipe not designed for a slow cooker. The only exception is when cooking rice or pasta. Then you'll want to increase the liquid. For every one cup of pasta, for example, you'll need two cups of water.
- Brown your meat in a skillet prior to placing it in the slow cooker. This will help reduce the fat in the finished dish. (Leaner meat does not need to be browned.)
- Don't lift the lid while cooking your dish. Doing so will release enough heat to cost you an additional 20 minutes of cooking time when cooking on low.
- Use whole herbs and spices. These produce more flavorful dishes. Ground spices can turn bitter with prolonged cooking.

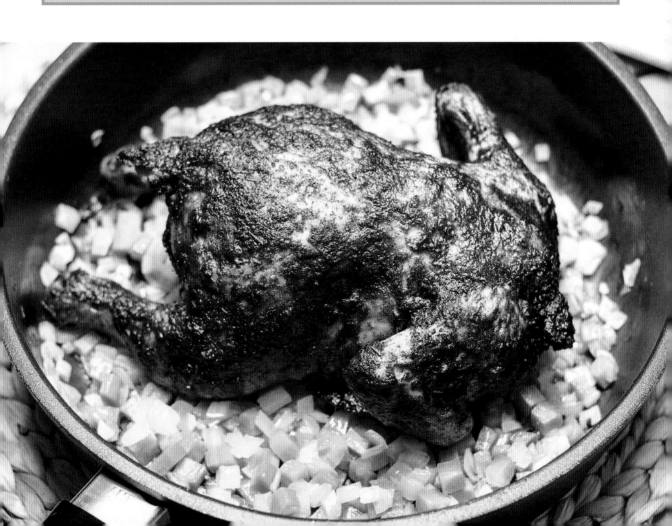

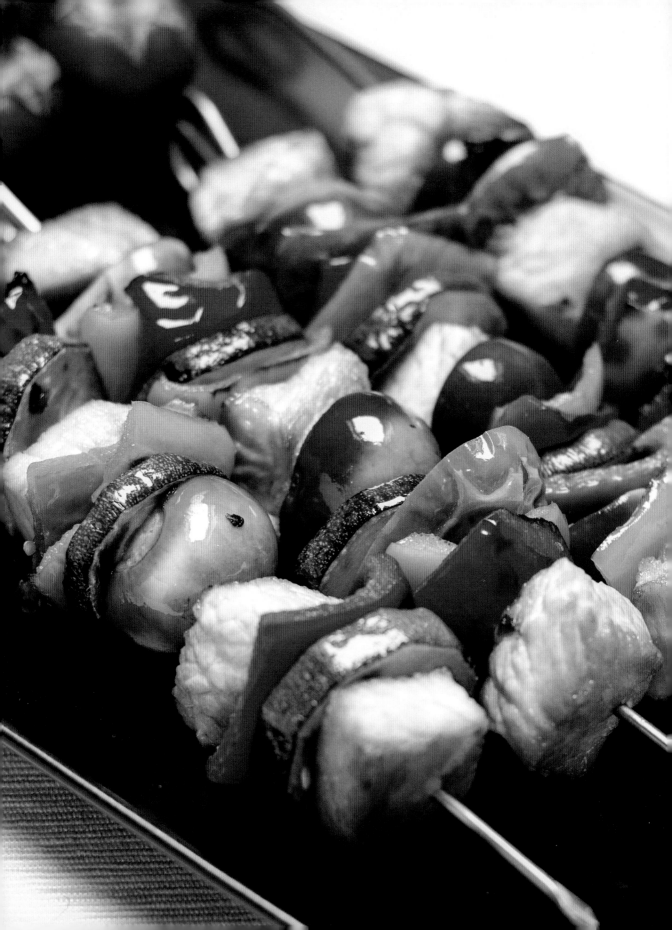

MEDITERRANEAN CHICKEN KABOBS

Kabobs are a Middle Eastern dish featuring pieces of meat, fish, or vegetables roasted or grilled on skewers. In this version, chicken and Mediterranean veggies are used to create this super-healthful dish. Served with pita bread (a fast fuel), this meal is as traditionally Mediterranean as it gets.

4 SERVINGS

1 large orange bell pepper

1 large green bell pepper

1 large red bell pepper

1 large zucchini

4 small baby eggplants

2 medium red onions

2 teaspoons lemon juice

1 tablespoon olive oil

1 garlic clove, crushed

1 tablespoon chopped fresh rosemary or
 1 teaspoon dried

2 skinless, boneless chicken breasts

4 whole-wheat pita breads

Cut bell peppers into even-sized pieces (not too small; otherwise the peppers will slide off the skewer). Cut zucchini into 1-inch slices. Cut baby eggplant in half and quarter them lengthwise. Cut onions into 6–8 wedges each. Place all vegetables in a large bowl.

In a small bowl, whisk together the lemon juice, olive oil, garlic, and rosemary. Season with salt and pepper. Pour the mixture over the vegetables and toss well to coat.

Preheat the grill on medium-high heat. Season chicken breasts with salt and pepper and grill for 5–10 minutes on each side, until cooked through. Cut into cubes.

Thread the vegetables and chicken onto the skewer and grill 2–4 minutes, until slightly charred. Serve the chicken and vegetables with pita bread.

NUTRITION PER SERVING | FAT: 10 GRAMS | CARBOHYDRATE: 46 GRAMS | PROTEIN: 37 GRAMS | TOTAL CALORIES: 422

THAI GREEN CHICKEN CURRY

This dish is Thai through and through, beginning with jasmine rice—a fast fuel—and including Thai curry paste. A mixture of chiles, lemongrass, and spices, Thai curry paste has no curry powder—it's not related to the Indian spice. You can find Thai curry paste in the Asian or international aisle of most big supermarkets.

4 SERVINGS

1 cup jasmine rice

1 tablespoon olive oil

3 garlic cloves, minced

1 cup diced onions

1 green bell pepper, diced

1 cup chopped skinless, boneless chicken breast

2 tablespoons Thai green curry paste (add more if you like)

1 tablespoon finely chopped ginger

One 14-ounce can lite (reduced-fat) coconut milk

1 small zucchini, cut into thick half-moons (about 1 cup)

Sugar

Fish sauce

1 cup chopped cilantro

Cook rice according to package directions and set aside.

Heat a large skillet over medium heat. Add oil, garlic, onions, and bell peppers and cook 3–5 minutes, until the vegetables are tender. Add chicken, green curry paste, and ginger and cook for 5 minutes more. Add coconut milk and 1/2 cup water and simmer over medium-low heat for an additional 5 minutes.

Add zucchini. Season with sugar to taste, fish sauce to taste, and salt and pepper. Cook 2–3 minutes more, until zucchini is tender. Serve over rice, garnished with cilantro.

NUTRITION PER SERVING | FAT: 12 GRAMS | CARBOHYDRATE: 18 GRAMS | PROTEIN: 14 GRAMS | TOTAL CALORIES: 236

CHICKEN AND SPINACH PIZZA

Here's a healthful, nutritious pizza so good you'll want to eat it every day. Its white sauce is what sets it apart. The pizza dough is a fast fuel.

8 SERVINGS

1 pound refrigerated whole-wheat pizza dough

1 tablespoon butter

2 garlic cloves, minced

2 tablespoons all-purpose flour

3/4 cup skim milk

1/2 cup grated Pecorino Romano cheese

1 tablespoon yellow cornmeal

11/2 cups shredded skinless, boneless rotisserie chicken breast

1/4 cup thinly sliced red onions

3/4 cup chopped spinach

1 tablespoon dried oregano

1 tablespoon chopped fresh chives

1 tablespoon chopped parsley

1 tablespoon chopped fresh basil

Preheat oven to 450 degrees. Place dough in a bowl, coat with cooking spray, and let stand, uncovered, 15 minutes.

In a small pot over medium heat, melt butter and add garlic. Cook for 30 seconds. Add flour and milk and cook, whisking constantly, until thick. Remove from heat and stir in the cheese. Season with salt and pepper.

Sprinkle the cornmeal on a baking sheet. Roll or pat the dough into a circle and transfer it to the cornmeal-covered baking sheet. Spread the cheese sauce on the dough, leaving a half inch border around the edge. Add the chicken, onions, and spinach, then sprinkle on the herbs. Bake for 15 minutes, or until the crust is golden.

NUTRITION PER SERVING | FAT: 8 GRAMS | CARBOHYDRATE: 23 GRAMS | PROTEIN: 20 GRAMS | TOTAL CALORIES: 244

CHICKEN AND VEGGIE PASTA

Pasta, a fast fuel, can be a healthful mealtime solution, especially if you ramp up the nutrients with lean protein like chicken and lots of vegetables. All of those extra vitamins, phytochemicals, and other goodies add up to high-powered food fuel. I've called for rotini—corkscrew-shaped pasta—but you could use any shape you like.

6 SERVINGS

2 skinless, boneless chicken breasts

4 tablespoons olive oil

1 teaspoon salt

1 tablespoon black pepper

3 tablespoons brown mustard

16 ounces whole-wheat rotini

4 ounces shredded Parmesan cheese

2 English cucumbers, diced

1/2 red bell pepper, thinly sliced

1/2 orange bell pepper, thinly sliced

1/2 yellow bell pepper, thinly sliced

1 small red onion, thinly sliced

1 cup torn fresh basil

Preheat grill to medium. Grill chicken 10 minutes on each side, until cooked through. Set aside to cool. Shred the chicken.

In a small bowl, combine olive oil, salt, black pepper, and mustard.

Cook the rotini according to package directions, and drain. Combine the pasta and the oil mixture, then add Parmesan cheese, chicken, cucumbers, peppers, and onions and toss gently. Garnish with the torn basil.

NUTRITION PER SERVING | FAT: 15 GRAMS | CARBOHYDRATE: 60 GRAMS | PROTEIN: 25 GRAMS | TOTAL CALORIES: 475

GNOCCHI AND SMOKED TURKEY SAUSAGE

Gnocchi are basically potato dumplings. The Italian word *gnocco* means "lump," but no matter how unattractive the shape might sound, gnocchi pair well with a whole host of ingredients. I've gone for a simple mixture of turkey sausage and veggies for a dish that's both delicious and really easy to make.

4 SERVINGS

1 pound gnocchi

One 13-ounce package smoked turkey sausage links, cut into 1/2-inch slices

3 garlic cloves, minced

1/2 cup chopped onions

1/2 cup cherry tomatoes, halved

4 cups tightly packed baby spinach

Cook gnocchi according to package instructions; drain and set aside.

Heat a large skillet over medium heat. Add sausage, garlic, onions, and tomatoes and cook 5 minutes, until the sausage is browned. Season with salt and pepper.

Add the gnocchi and cook 2–3 minutes, until heated through. Add spinach and cook until just wilted.

NUTRITION PER SERVING FAT: 10 GRAMS CARBOHYDRATE: 25 GRAMS PROTEIN: 19 GRAMS TOTAL CALORIES: 266

TURKEY PICADILLO

Think of this dish as a sort of Cuban sloppy Joe, though you won't be serving the meat mixture on buns; it pairs much better with brown rice, a fast fuel. This savory and sweet Latin American dish is usually made with ground beef, but I decided to try it with ground turkey, and the results are fantastic. The leftover prepared meat stores well and is easy to heat up for another meal later in the week.

6 SERVINGS

2 cups brown rice

2 tablespoons olive oil

1 pound ground turkey

1 large yellow onion, chopped

1 green bell pepper, chopped

4 garlic cloves, minced

2 bay leaves

1/2 cup white wine

One 8-ounce can tomato sauce

1/3 cup green olives, chopped

1/3 cup raisins

1 tablespoon capers

1/2 teaspoon cayenne, or to taste

1/4 teaspoon dried oregano

2 teaspoons ground cumin

1 tablespoon chopped parsley

Prepare brown rice according to package directions and set aside.

Heat 1 tablespoon oil in a large skillet over medium-high heat. Add turkey and cook, stirring, until browned. Season with salt and pepper. Remove turkey and discard any excess grease.

Heat the same skillet over medium heat and add the remaining 1 tablespoon olive oil, the onions, bell peppers, garlic, and bay leaves. Cook 5 minutes, until onions are soft. Stir in the turkey mixture, wine, tomato sauce, olives, raisins, capers, cayenne, oregano, and cumin and simmer 15 minutes. Serve with the brown rice and garnish with parsley.

NUTRITION PER SERVING | FAT: 6 GRAMS | CARBOHYDRATE: 30 GRAMS | PROTEIN: 18 GRAMS | TOTAL CALORIES: 246

LOW-FAT LASAGNA

I adore lasagna—how could you not love something that celebrates the culinary trio of pasta, cheese, and tomatoes?—but it can be quite fattening. Here's a fat- and calorie-downsized version of this classic Italian dish that doesn't sacrifice flavor. This recipe will serve a crowd, or you can eat it one serving at a time—just store the leftovers in the fridge, covered.

12 SERVINGS

1 pound whole-wheat lasagna noodles

1 tablespoon olive oil

1 pound ground turkey

3/4 cup chopped onions

3 garlic cloves, minced

One 46-ounce jar low-sugar or low-carbohydrate pasta sauce

1/2 teaspoon fennel seeds

1 teaspoon Italian seasoning

16 ounces part-skim ricotta

1/2 cup chopped parsley

1 large egg

12 ounces shredded fat-free mozzarella

3/4 cup grated Parmesan cheese

Preheat oven to 375 degrees. Cook noodles al dente according to package directions, drain, and set aside. Don't overcook the noodles, or they will fall apart as you are building this dish.

Heat a large skillet over medium heat. Add the oil, turkey, onions, and garlic and cook for 15 minutes, until browned. Stir in the pasta sauce, fennel seeds, and Italian seasoning. Simmer uncovered for about 15 minutes, stirring occasionally. Season with salt and pepper.

In a medium bowl, combine the ricotta, parsley, and egg.

Spread 11/2 cups turkey mixture in bottom of 9-by-13-inch baking dish. Layer noodles to completely cover the sauce. Spread half the ricotta mixture over the noodles, then top with a third of the mozzarella cheese and sprinkle with 1/4 cup Parmesan. Repeat layers and top with remaining mozzarella and Parmesan cheese. Cover with aluminum foil. Make sure the foil does not touch the cheese.

Bake 25 minutes, until the sauce is hot and the cheese is melted. Remove foil and bake 10–15 minutes more, until the cheese is lightly browned. Let cool for 10–15 minutes before serving.

NUTRITION PER SERVING | FAT: 9 GRAMS | CARBOHYDRATE: 43 GRAMS | PROTEIN: 23 GRAMS | TOTAL CALORIES: 345

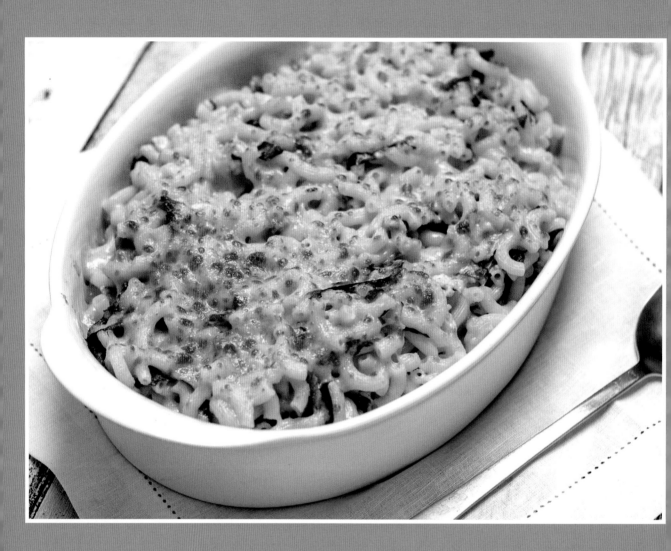

CHEESEBURGER MACARONI

Here's a twist on a comfort food that never goes out of style: warm and gooey macaroni and cheese. I've powered it up with the addition of lean ground turkey breast and turned it into a high-protein meal. This recipe also uses a variety of low-fat dairy foods, along with veggies and whole-wheat elbow pasta (a fast fuel)—a winning and healthful combination.

6 SERVINGS

8 ounces whole-wheat elbow pasta

1/4 cup low-fat milk

2 cups shredded reduced-fat sharp cheddar cheese

2/3 cup plain low-fat Greek yogurt

1/4 teaspoon garlic powder

1/4 teaspoon onion powder

1/2 cup chopped onions

3 tablespoons minced garlic

1 pound ground turkey

2 cups chopped spinach

1/2 cup chopped green bell peppers

1 tomato, chopped

1/2 cup chopped scallions

Preheat oven to 400 degrees.

Cook pasta according to package directions; drain and return pasta to pot. Add milk, 13/4 cups cheese, yogurt, garlic powder, and onion powder, stirring until cheese is melted and pasta is completely coated.

Coat a large skillet with cooking spray and heat over medium heat. Sauté onions and garlic until onions are translucent. Add turkey, spinach, and bell peppers and cook until meat is no longer pink. Season with salt and pepper.

Add meat mixture and tomatoes to the pasta and cheese and mix well. Coat a 9-by-13-inch baking dish with cooking spray and transfer meat and pasta mixture into dish. Sprinkle the rest of the cheese on top. Bake 15 minutes, until cheese is melted and lightly brown. Sprinkle with scallions.

NUTRITION PER SERVING | FAT: 9 GRAMS | CARBOHYDRATE: 13 GRAMS | PROTEIN: 32 GRAMS | TOTAL CALORIES: 270

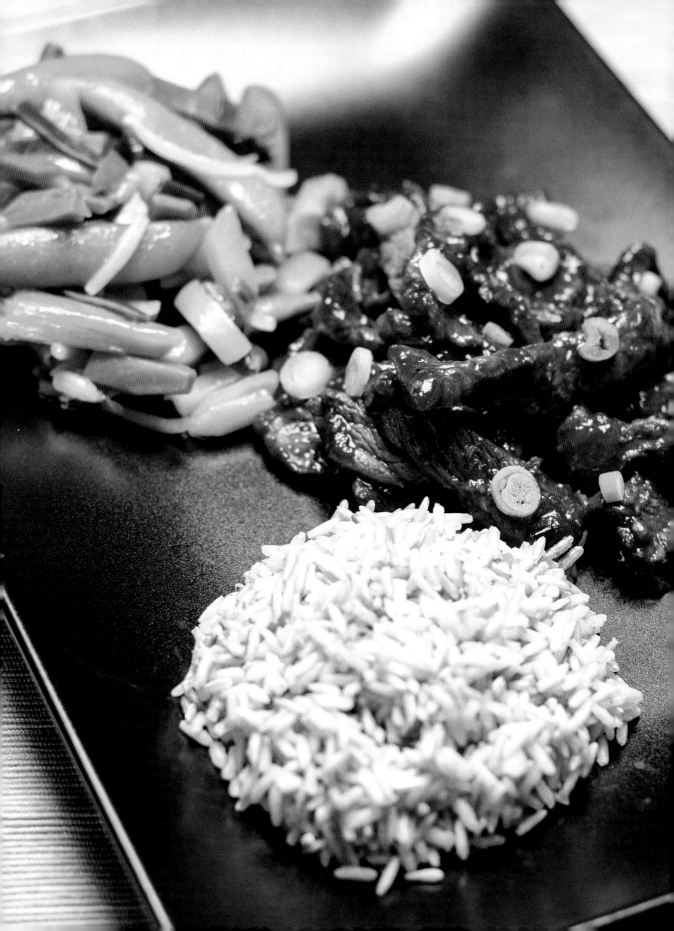

GINGER BEEF

While this dish is a staple on many Asian menus, you can now whip it up easily at home without worrying about hidden fat, sugars, or additives that are often lurking in restaurant fare. Use fresh ginger and garlic to spice up this dish. Brown rice is a fast fuel.

4 SERVINGS

2 cups brown rice

2 teaspoons cornstarch

16 ounces tri-tip or sirloin steak, thinly sliced (see sidebar)

2 tablespoons grated ginger

1/4 cup low-sodium soy sauce

1/8 teaspoon black pepper

1 tablespoon brown mustard

1 tablespoon olive oil

1/2 red onion, chopped

3 garlic cloves, minced

One 12-ounce package frozen Asian vegetables, thawed

2 scallions, chopped

Cook the brown rice according to package directions and set aside. In a small bowl, mix cornstarch with a little water and whisk until smooth; set aside.

Combine the beef, ginger, soy sauce, pepper, and mustard, and marinate for about 20 minutes.

Heat a large skillet over high heat. Add olive oil, onions, and garlic. Cook, stirring, 2–3 minutes, until onions have softened. Add the beef and stir-fry 2–3 minutes more.

Add Asian vegetables and stir-fry 2–3 minutes. Add the cornstarch mixture to the meat and vegetables and stir until thickened.

Serve over the rice and sprinkle scallions on top.

HOO-YA

SLICING MEAT THINLY

Sometimes raw beef can be tough to slice. Here's a tip I've found invaluable for neatly slicing meat: place the steak in the freezer for 10–15 minutes before you attempt to slice it. You'll be able to get much thinner, more even slices.

NUTRITION PER SERVING | FAT: 11 GRAMS | CARBOHYDRATE: 32 GRAMS | PROTEIN: 28 GRAMS | TOTAL CALORIES: 339

EASY LINGUINE WITH MEAT SAUCE

Linguine (the name means "little tongues" in Italian) is usually served with seafood or pesto. It holds up just as well to a red meat sauce, my version of which is quick, flavorful, and loaded with onions and bell peppers to fill you up. Like all pastas, linguine is a fast fuel.

4 SERVINGS

16 ounces whole-wheat linguine

½ pound lean ground beef

1 small green bell pepper, diced

2 cups chopped onions

1 tablespoon minced garlic

1 teaspoon dried oregano

3 tablespoons tomato paste

One 14.5-ounce can diced tomatoes

¼ cup shaved Parmigiano-Reggiano cheese

2 tablespoons chopped parsley

Cook pasta according to package directions. Drain and set aside.

While the pasta cooks, heat a large skillet over medium-high heat. Cook beef, bell peppers, onions, garlic, and oregano 5 minutes, until beef is browned. Season with salt and pepper.

Stir in tomato paste and diced tomatoes. Bring to a boil, then reduce heat to medium-low and cook for another 3 minutes, until sauce thickens. Serve pasta topped with meat sauce and garnished with cheese and parsley.

| NUTRITION PER SERVING | FAT: 7 GRAMS | CARBOHYDRATE: 62 GRAMS | PROTEIN: 23 GRAMS | TOTAL CALORIES: 402 |

SLOW COOKER INDIAN LAMB CURRY

When I get super-busy, I drag out my slow cooker. It takes the top prize for making a busy cook's life a little less hectic—and a majority of the population agrees with me. Approximately 83 percent of families own one, according to *Consumer Reports*. This recipe cooks up a classic lamb stew, with an Indian twist for extra flavor, and pairs it with brown rice, a fast fuel.

8 SERVINGS

2 pounds lamb, trimmed of excess fat and cut into 1-inch cubes
One 14.5-ounce can diced tomatoes
2 tablespoons all-purpose flour
2 teaspoons mustard seeds
4 garlic cloves, minced
2 cups finely chopped white onions
½ cup chopped carrots

2 tablespoons grated ginger
2 teaspoons garam masala (see sidebar)
2 teaspoons ground cumin
½ teaspoon salt
¼ teaspoon crushed red pepper
4 cups cooked brown rice
½ cup plain fat-free yogurt
½ cup chopped cilantro

Sauté lamb in a large nonstick skillet over medium-high heat for 5 minutes, until browned. Place lamb in a 4-quart slow cooker.

Drain the canned tomatoes, reserving the juice. Add flour to tomato juice and whisk until smooth. Add to the slow cooker the tomatoes, tomato juice mixture, mustard seeds, garlic, onions, carrots, ginger, garam masala, cumin, salt, and crushed red pepper. Cover and cook on low for 6–8 hours, until lamb is tender. Serve lamb curry over rice and top with yogurt and cilantro.

HOO-YA

GARAM MASALA

If you're new to Indian cooking, let me introduce you to garam masala, a blend of spices used in this cuisine. In Hindi, *garam* means "warm" and *masala* means "blend of spices." Typically, those spices include coriander seeds, cumin, cayenne pepper, turmeric, ginger, black pepper, cardamom, cloves, and cinnamon.

Garam masala is used in many Indian dishes. You can find it in the spice section of most grocery stores.

NUTRITION PER SERVING | FAT: 16 GRAMS | CARBOHYDRATE: 35 GRAMS | PROTEIN: 42 GRAMS | TOTAL CALORIES: 452

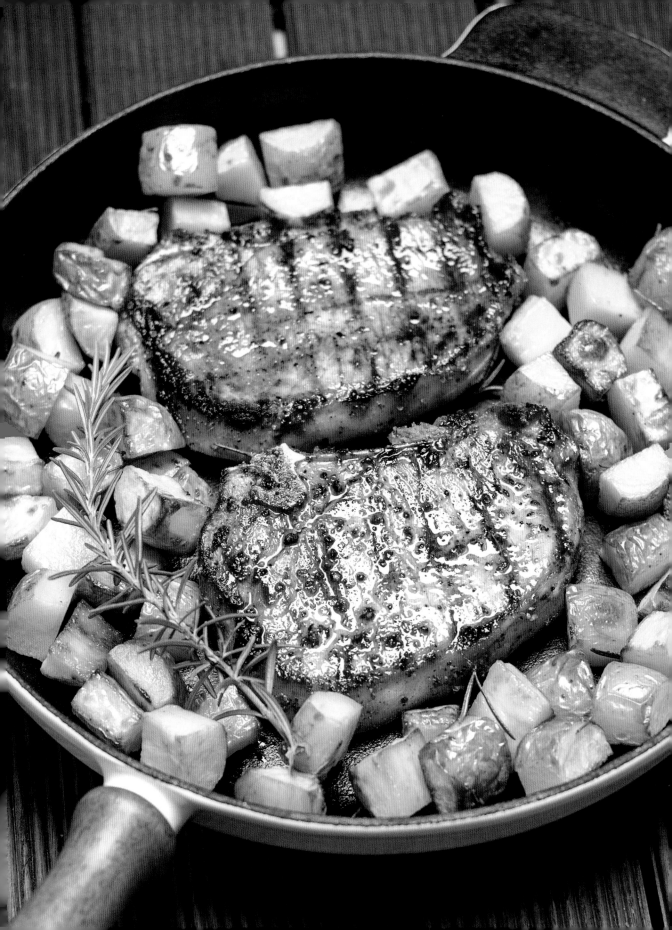

FIVE-SPICE PORK CHOPS

Give me a thick, grilled pork chop, spiced and cooked to a perfect pinkness, with a great side dish, and I'm in hog heaven. With this recipe, that side dish is roasted potatoes (a fast fuel) with rosemary, an herb that takes spuds to new levels of goodness. The seasoning for the pork is five-spice powder, which can be found in the Asian section of most supermarkets.

4 SERVINGS

2 tablespoons five-spice powder

1 teaspoon black pepper

3 tablespoons fish sauce

2 tablespoons sugar

2 tablespoons brown mustard

4 pork loin chops

2 cups fingerling potatoes

2 tablespoons olive oil

1 tablespoon coarse Himalayan salt

1/2 bunch rosemary

Preheat oven to 350 degrees.

Combine five-spice powder blend, pepper, fish sauce, sugar, mustard, and 1/4 cup water in a small bowl and blend well. Pour over pork chops and let marinate for about an hour.

Wash and dry the potatoes and cut them in cubes. Toss with olive oil, salt, and rosemary. Roast 10–15 minutes, or until potatoes are tender.

Preheat grill to medium. Grill pork chops about 7 minutes on each side, until cooked thoroughly. Make sure to keep an eye on the pork chops so that they do not become too dry. Serve the chops with the roasted potatoes.

NUTRITION PER SERVING | FAT: 10 GRAMS | CARBOHYDRATE: 20 GRAMS | PROTEIN: 25 GRAMS | TOTAL CALORIES: 289

LIGHT MEATLESS SPAGHETTI

V

When you think of spaghetti the word "light" isn't usually what comes to mind, but it's not the pasta itself that is heavy; it's the traditional pairing with cheese and meat. In this recipe, I've dispensed with both. As a stand-in for meat, I've used a textured vegetable protein that does a pretty good imitation of ground beef. You don't have to cook the sauce in a slow cooker—cooking time would be 15–20 minutes on the stovetop—but if you use a slow cooker, you'll have a warm meal waiting for you when you get home!

6 SERVINGS

1 tablespoon olive oil

3 garlic cloves, minced

½ cup chopped onions

⅔ cup chopped carrots

⅔ cup chopped celery

3 cups imitation ground meat (textured vegetable protein)

½ teaspoon nutmeg

¼ cup dry white wine

1½ cups canned plum tomatoes, chopped; reserve juice

16 ounces whole-wheat pasta

½ cup half-and-half

Basil for garnish

Heat a large skillet over medium-high heat. Add oil, garlic, onions, carrots, and celery and cook 2 minutes. Add the imitation ground meat and cook for another 2 minutes. Season with salt and pepper, then transfer to slow cooker.

Add the rest of the ingredients, except the pasta, the half-and-half, and the basil, to the slow cooker. Cover and cook on low for 8 hours or on high for 4 hours.

When ready to serve, cook the pasta according to package directions and drain. Stir the half-and-half into the sauce. Pour the sauce over the pasta and garnish with basil.

NUTRITION PER SERVING	FAT: 8 GRAMS	CARBOHYDRATE: 60 GRAMS	PROTEIN: 19 GRAMS	TOTAL CALORIES: 388

VEGGIE ENCHILADAS

Mexican food lends itself very well to vegetarian entrées thanks to the abundance of beans, veggies, and other healthful fuels. This recipe, with its meaty-tasting black beans, is an example of what I'm talking about. The flavors of Mexico take over deliciously, and you won't even miss the meat.

8 SERVINGS

1 tablespoon olive oil

1 green bell pepper, sliced

1 cup corn kernels

1 large portobello mushroom, sliced

1 red onion, thinly sliced

One 15-ounce can black beans, rinsed and drained

1 teaspoon ground cumin

8 whole-wheat tortillas

2 cups canned enchilada sauce

2 cups shredded reduced-fat Mexican-blend cheese

¼ cup low-fat sour cream

½ cup chopped cilantro

Cholula Hot Sauce

Preheat oven to 350 degrees. Coat a baking dish with cooking spray.

In a large skillet, heat oil and cook the bell peppers, corn, mushrooms, and onions until tender. Add the beans and cumin. Season with salt and pepper. Spoon ⅛ of the bean mixture in the center of each tortilla, roll up, and place seam side down in the baking dish. Repeat. Cover the rolled tortillas with the enchilada sauce and top with cheese.

Bake 20–30 minutes, until cheese is melted and sauce is bubbling. Garnish with sour cream, cilantro, and Cholula Hot Sauce.

HOO-YA

CHOLULA HOT SAUCE

If you love hot sauce, here's one to try: Cholula Hot Sauce (choe-LOO-la). It's a blend of red peppers, piquin peppers, and spices. This hot pepper sauce was named after a 2,500-year-old city in Mexico, the oldest inhabited city in North America. You can purchase it in most supermarkets. The manufacturer says it's delicious on everything but peanut butter!

NUTRITION PER SERVING | FAT: 8 GRAMS | CARBOHYDRATE: 39 GRAMS | PROTEIN: 12 GRAMS | TOTAL CALORIES: 27

QUINOA AND TURKEY CHORIZO-STUFFED CHILES

The poblano chile, sometimes called a pasilla, is large, shiny, black-green in color, and mild. It is perfect for stuffing because of its size and fleshy texture. Do not remove the stem, because it serves as a natural handle. Quinoa is the fast fuel.

4 SERVINGS

1 cup quinoa

4 large poblano chiles

½ tablespoon olive oil

½ cup chopped green bell peppers

¼ cup diced onions

12 ounces turkey chorizo, crumbled and cooked

½ cup queso fresco

1 cup chopped cilantro

1 thinly sliced red jalapeño

Preheat the oven to 400 degrees.

Cook quinoa according to package directions.

Cut a slit on one side of each chile, keeping the stem and tip intact. Remove and discard the seeds.

In a small skillet, heat oil and sauté bell peppers and onions until soft.

In a large bowl, combine the bell pepper and onion mixture with the chorizo, quinoa, queso fresco (reserve a little for topping), and ½ cup cilantro. Season with salt and pepper.

Stuff the filling into the chiles and place them on a baking sheet. Roast until the chiles are tender and the filling is browned, about 25 minutes.

Top with the sliced jalapeño, the remaining cheese, and the remaining cilantro.

NUTRITION PER SERVING | FAT: 17 GRAMS | CARBOHYDRATE: 38 GRAMS | PROTEIN: 30 GRAMS | TOTAL CALORIES: 425

HOO-YA

QUINOA, THE HIGH-PROTEIN CARB

I've started enjoying quinoa (pronounced KEEN-wa) in more of my meals because it is gluten-free, so easy to digest, and high in fiber. Most people think quinoa is a grain, but it is actually an herb. What also differentiates it from grains is that it is a complete protein. That means it contains all eight essential amino acids. Quinoa is also loaded with more minerals than most grains, including calcium, phosphorus, magnesium, potassium, iron, and zinc.

Quinoa is easy to cook, too. You just boil it in water. When the tiny grains turn into little circles, it's done—a process that takes less than 20 minutes.

Quinoa is versatile. Enjoy it as a cereal in the morning with milk and fruit. Serve it as a side dish, flavored with herbs such as garlic or dill, or mix it with your favorite cooked veggies.

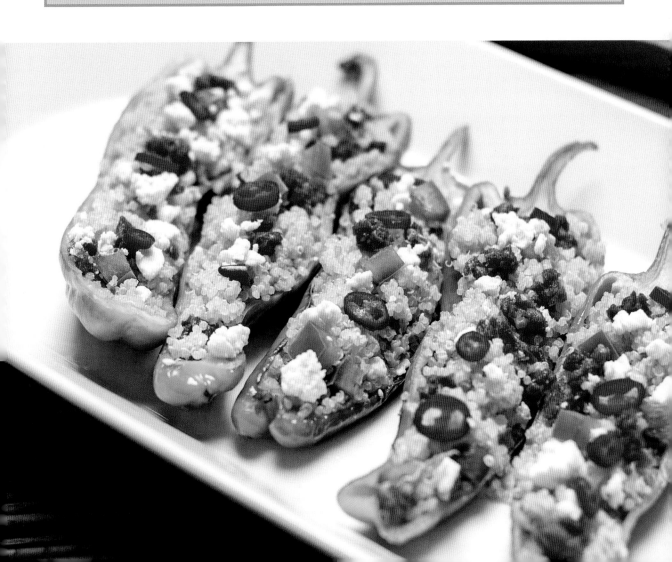

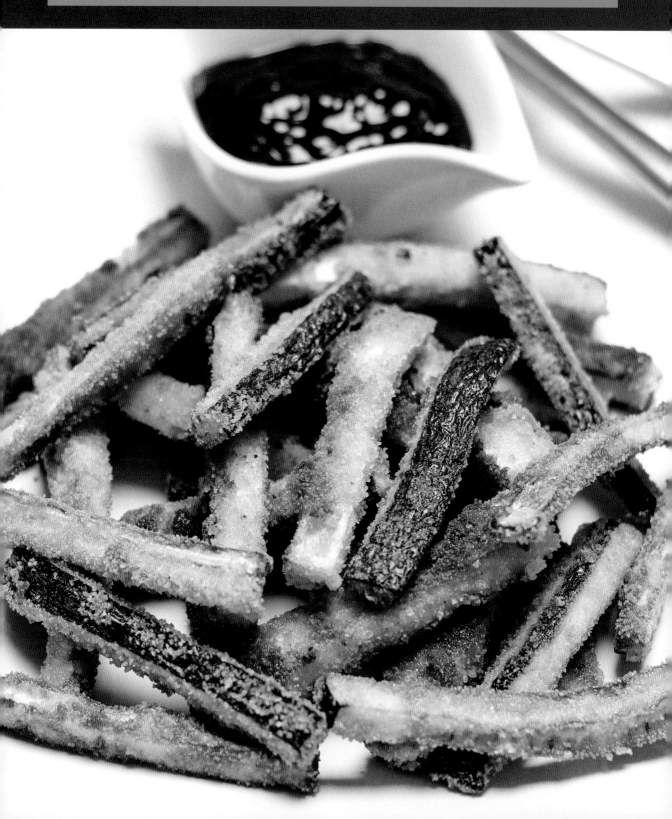

ZUCCHINI FRIES

When you're craving french fries, these are a more healthful alternative. Panko (Japanese-style bread crumbs), a fast fuel, give the fries their crunch.

4 SERVINGS

2 large eggs

2 cups panko (Japanese-style bread crumbs)

1 teaspoon garlic powder

1 tablespoon grated Parmesan cheese

4 large zucchini, cut lengthwise into "fries" 3–4 inches long

Preheat oven to 375 degrees. Coat 2 baking sheets with cooking spray.

In a small bowl, beat the eggs. In another small bowl, combine the bread crumbs, garlic powder, and cheese; season with salt and pepper.

Dip the zucchini strips in the beaten eggs. Roll each strip in the bread crumb mixture, making sure the zucchini is completely covered with bread crumbs. Place the coated zucchini strips on baking sheets.

Bake the zucchini 10–15 minutes. Turn the zucchini over and bake another 10–15 minutes, until golden brown.

NUTRITION PER SERVING | FAT: 3 GRAMS | CARBOHYDRATE: 27 GRAMS | PROTEIN: 8 GRAMS | TOTAL CALORIES: 263

HOW TO MAKE HOMEMADE KETCHUP

Ketchup is notoriously high in sugar, and the reduced-sugar versions are made with artificial sweeteners. If you're trying to avoid both, the solution is to make your own ketchup. It's easy to do. Here's a recipe to get you started.

MARK'S EASY HOMEMADE KETCHUP

MAKES APPROXIMATELY 11/2 CUPS

One 6-ounce can tomato paste

2 tablespoons apple cider vinegar

¼ teaspoon dry mustard

¾ teaspoon salt

¾ teaspoon onion powder

¼ teaspoon cinnamon

Optional for sweetness: a pinch of stevia

Combine all the ingredients with ⅓ cup water and whisk well to combine. Refrigerate overnight to let the flavors develop. Use as you would any commercial brand of ketchup.

BAKED SALMON FISH STICKS

Even though they taste good, packaged fish sticks are often loaded with preservatives. Here's a recipe that will give you all the great taste of fish sticks and is super-healthful, too. They make a great post-workout revitalizer and can also be served as a lunch or dinner entrée.

4 SERVINGS

1 pound wild salmon fillet
1 cup seasoned bread crumbs
½ teaspoon lemon pepper seasoning

½ teaspoon paprika
½ cup all-purpose flour
2 egg whites, beaten

Preheat oven to 350 degrees. Coat a baking sheet with cooking spray.

Cut salmon into strips ½ inch wide by 4 inches long.

In a shallow bowl, mix bread crumbs, lemon pepper seasoning, and paprika. Place flour in a second shallow bowl and the egg whites in a third. Dip fish into the flour and then the egg mixture before coating with the bread crumbs. Make sure to coat both sides. Place on baking sheet. Bake 10–15 minutes, until fish is golden brown.

NUTRITION PER SERVING | FAT: 11 GRAMS | CARBOHYDRATE: 32 GRAMS | PROTEIN: 34 GRAMS | TOTAL CALORIES: 363

ALMOND BUTTER AND JELLY RICE CAKES

You can fix these in no time at all and have them ready to eat after you finish your workout. Each sandwich is loaded with fast fuel in the form of strawberries and rice cakes to replenish the energy in your muscles after exercising.

4 SERVINGS

1 cup strawberries

1 tablespoon chia seeds

1 tablespoon agave syrup

4 tablespoons almond butter

8 large brown rice cakes

In a small bowl, combine the strawberries, chia seeds, agave, and 1 tablespoon water. Smash the mixture with a fork until it has the consistency of jam.

Spread almond butter on top of one rice cake and top with strawberry-chia jam. Sandwich with another rice cake. Continue this with the remaining rice cakes.

NUTRITION PER SERVING | FAT: 9 GRAMS | CARBOHYDRATE: 40 GRAMS | PROTEIN: 6 GRAMS | TOTAL CALORIES: 265

Chapter 4

Slow-Fuel Meals

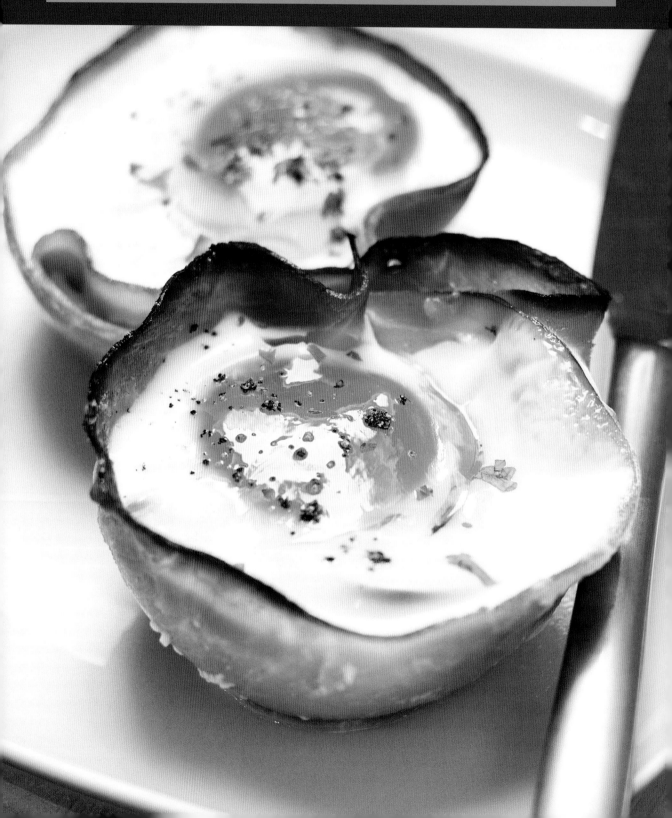

BREAKFAST CUPS

I don't know which is more fun: making these breakfast gems or eating them. Here's a recipe with all the nutritional goodness of a veggie omelet, but without the messy flipping!

12 SERVINGS

12 thin slices Canadian bacon
½ cup shredded reduced-fat cheddar cheese
½ cup sliced button mushrooms
12 large eggs

6 grape tomatoes, halved
Garlic powder
¼ cup parsley, minced

Preheat oven to 350 degrees. Coat a 12-cup muffin tin with cooking spray.

Drape one Canadian bacon slice in each of the cups in the muffin tin. Divide the cheese among the cups, followed by the mushrooms. Carefully crack an egg in each cup, then place a tomato half on top. Sprinkle them with garlic powder to taste, and season with salt and pepper.

Bake for 20 minutes, or until eggs are set. Garnish with parsley.

HOO-YA

COOKING IN BULK

With recipes like my Breakfast Cups, you're going to have leftovers—and that's a good thing. You can pop the extra cups in the freezer and heat them up later.

In fact, many of my recipes make more than 1 or 2 servings. Stash those leftovers in the freezer for a fast, easy meal in the future. Cooking in bulk is smart cooking—and great for people on the go.

NUTRITION PER SERVING | FAT: 8 GRAMS | CARBOHYDRATE: 3 GRAMS | PROTEIN: 19 GRAMS | TOTAL CALORIES: 160

EGG AND SQUASH SKILLET

Hash browns are a delicious but greasy and fattening potato dish. Try this easy-to-make recipe that substitutes squash and veggies for the potatoes. I'll bet you won't miss the traditional preparation at all! Because this makes 6 servings, you can eat it every morning for a week.

6 SERVINGS

6 zucchini or yellow squash

8 slices Canadian bacon, diced

1 tablespoon olive oil

1/2 cup chopped onions

4 scallions, thinly sliced

1 jalapeño, seeded and minced

3 tablespoons chopped parsley

1/4 teaspoon nutmeg

6 large eggs

1/2 cup shredded reduced-fat sharp cheddar cheese

Preheat oven to 375 degrees.

Using the large holes of a box grater, grate the squash into a colander. Sprinkle the squash with salt and let it drain in the sink for 30 minutes. Squeeze the squash to remove as much liquid as possible.

In a large ovenproof skillet, cook the Canadian bacon and set aside. Heat the olive oil in the same skillet over medium-high heat. Add the onions, half the scallions, and the jalapeños and cook until the onions are soft. Add the squash, parsley, and nutmeg, season with salt and pepper, and cook until the mixture is slightly dry. Add the Canadian bacon and spread the mixture evenly in the skillet.

Make six 3-inch indentations in the mixture with the back of a spoon, then crack an egg into each indentation. Sprinkle the cheese over the mixture and season with salt and pepper. Transfer the skillet to the oven and bake until eggs are set, about 10 minutes. Sprinkle the rest of the scallions over the top before serving.

| NUTRITION PER SERVING | FAT: 10 GRAMS | CARBOHYDRATE: 14 GRAMS | PROTEIN: 18 GRAMS | TOTAL CALORIES: 218 |

EGGS IN A NEST

Portobello mushrooms are so large and meaty that they work perfectly as a "nest" for cooked eggs. Here's a filling slow-fuel breakfast that will get your day started off right. You won't even miss your toast or cereal.

1 SERVING

2 portobello mushroom caps, stems removed

2 large eggs

1 teaspoon garlic powder

1 tablespoon olive oil

1 cup tightly packed baby spinach

2 tomato slices

1 tablespoon goat cheese

Preheat oven to 400 degrees.

Coat a baking sheet with cooking spray. Place the mushrooms on the sheet and cook 5–7 minutes on each side. Turn and cook an additional 5–7 minutes, until any liquid has evaporated.

Coat a skillet with cooking spray and heat over medium-high heat. Crack 2 eggs into the pan and cook until the egg whites are set. Sprinkle the eggs with garlic powder and season with salt and pepper. When the eggs are cooked to your liking, remove them from the pan and set aside. In the same pan, add oil and sauté the spinach for 2 minutes, until wilted.

Arrange the spinach on a plate. Top with the mushrooms, tomato slices, and eggs, and sprinkle goat cheese on top.

NUTRITION PER SERVING | FAT: 15 GRAMS | CARBOHYDRATE: 18 GRAMS | PROTEIN: 20 GRAMS | TOTAL CALORIES: 287

BACON SCRAMBLED OVER ASPARAGUS

Asparagus in the morning? Sure! Why not start your day with a blast of health benefits? Research suggests that eating asparagus may help promote heart health, protect your liver, act as a cleansing diuretic, and help manage diabetes. Plus, this slow-fuel veggie is just downright delicious.

4 SERVINGS

11/2 pounds asparagus, hard ends trimmed

2 tablespoons olive oil

6 large eggs

3 tablespoons low-fat milk

1 cup sliced Canadian bacon, diced

1 teaspoon garlic powder

2 tablespoons butter

1/4 cup thinly sliced scallions

Preheat oven to 425 degrees and coat a baking sheet with cooking spray.

Place asparagus on the baking sheet. Drizzle with the oil and season with salt and pepper. Bake for 15 minutes, until tips start to get crisp. Transfer to a plate.

Beat the eggs in a large bowl and stir in milk, bacon, and garlic powder; season with salt and pepper. Heat a large pan and melt the butter over medium-high heat. Add egg mixture and stir gently until cooked and soft; be careful not to overcook.

Spoon scrambled eggs over asparagus and garnish with scallions.

NUTRITION PER SERVING | FAT: 15 GRAMS | CARBOHYDRATE: 7 GRAMS | PROTEIN: 15 GRAMS | TOTAL CALORIES: 223

BAKED BROCCOLI AND CHEDDAR FRITTATA

If you like omelets, you'll love the easier-to-make frittata. A frittata is very similar to an omelet; it's also like a crustless quiche that's baked in a skillet. And you don't have to worry about folding it!

4 SERVINGS

5 large eggs

5 egg whites

1 tablespoon olive oil

1 small onion, thinly sliced

2 cups frozen chopped broccoli, thawed

1/4 teaspoon garlic powder

1/2 cup shredded reduced-fat sharp cheddar cheese

Preheat oven to 400 degrees. Position a rack in the middle of the oven.

Whisk eggs and egg whites with 2 tablespoons water in a large bowl; set aside.

Heat oil in a large ovenproof nonstick skillet over medium heat. Add onions and cook 3 minutes, until they begin to soften. Add broccoli and garlic powder, season with salt and pepper, and cook 2 minutes more.

Pour eggs over vegetables, covering them evenly. Reduce the heat to medium-low, cover, and let cook until the egg mixture has set around the edges of the pan.

Sprinkle the egg mixture with cheese and transfer the pan to the oven. Bake 1–2 minutes, until the frittata is golden brown and puffed; be careful not to overcook. Transfer frittata to a cutting board and cut into 4 pieces.

NUTRITION PER SERVING | FAT: 13 GRAMS | CARBOHYDRATE: 5 GRAMS | PROTEIN: 19 GRAMS | TOTAL CALORIES: 213

SMOKED GOUDA AND VEGGIE FRITTATA

Though I love them, there's more to life than scrambled eggs. So why not start your morning with this vegetable frittata? This slow-fuel breakfast is so filling that there's no way you'll go hungry. The addition of smoked Gouda gives this dish an almost bacon-y flavor that's hard to resist.

4 SERVINGS

2 large eggs

4 large egg whites

1 teaspoon finely chopped fresh rosemary

1/2 cup shredded smoked Gouda

1 tablespoon olive oil

1/3 cup sliced onions

1/3 cup sliced red bell peppers

1/2 cup frozen peas, thawed

1 cup sliced mushrooms

4 cups torn baby spinach

Preheat oven to 350 degrees.

In a large bowl, beat the eggs and egg whites. Add rosemary and 1/4 cup smoked Gouda. Season with salt and pepper. Set aside.

Heat a large skillet over medium-high heat. Add oil and onions and cook for 2 minutes. Add the bell peppers, peas, and mushrooms and cook for 2 minutes more. Add the spinach and cook for another minute. Pour the veggie mixture into the eggs and mix well.

Coat a round cake pan with cooking spray. Pour egg-veggie mixture into the pan. Top with the remaining cheese and bake for 30 minutes, until eggs are set. Cut into 4 wedges and serve.

NUTRITION PER SERVING | FAT: 13 GRAMS | CARBOHYDRATE: 7 GRAMS | PROTEIN: 15 GRAMS | TOTAL CALORIES: 205

ATHLETIC OMELET

Egg-white omelets are a favorite of athletes looking to eat a lot of protein and to cut a few caloric corners. Egg whites themselves have a slightly bland flavor, but this makes them a great partner for stronger-tasting ingredients—Canadian bacon, cheese, and onions, for example, as I've included in this recipe.

1 SERVING

1 tablespoon diced onions
2 slices Canadian bacon, diced
1/4 cup sliced button mushrooms
1/4 cup diced tomatoes

1/4 cup diced green bell peppers
4 egg whites
1/4 cup shredded reduced-fat cheddar cheese
Cilantro for garnish

Coat a large skillet with cooking spray and heat over medium-high heat. Cook onions, bacon, mushrooms, tomatoes, and bell peppers 2–3 minutes, until peppers are tender. Season with salt and pepper and set aside.

Add more cooking spray to the skillet. Beat the egg whites well and pour into the pan. Cook until egg is nearly set. Add the bacon-veggie mixture to one half of the omelet and top with cheese. Flip the other side of the omelet over the bacon-veggie-cheese mixture and cook for 1–2 minutes more, until cheese has melted. Garnish with cilantro.

NUTRITION PER SERVING	FAT: 6 GRAMS	CARBOHYDRATE: 12 GRAMS	PROTEIN: 46 GRAMS	TOTAL CALORIES: 286

SMOKED HAM AND SPINACH QUICHE

Quiche is among the easiest and tastiest meals to make. All you do is mix an assortment of flavorful ingredients together with eggs, pour into a dish, and bake. My mouthwatering quiche bypasses the usual dough and is made crustless in a pie pan spritzed with cooking spray. You won't even miss the crust.

6 SERVINGS

¾ cup cubed smoked turkey ham

½ cup chopped onions

½ cup chopped red bell peppers

½ cup chopped button mushrooms

¾ cup shredded Swiss cheese

¼ cup shredded reduced-fat cheddar cheese

1 cup tightly packed baby spinach

1 cup fat-free cottage cheese

½ cup milk

2 large eggs

2 egg whites

½ cup all-purpose flour

1 teaspoon baking powder

Preheat oven to 350 degrees.

Coat a skillet with cooking spray and heat over medium-high heat. Add ham, onions, bell peppers, and mushrooms and sauté 3–4 minutes. Season with pepper.

Coat a 9-inch pie plate with cooking spray. Sprinkle with ¼ cup Swiss cheese and add the ham mixture.

In a large bowl, combine the remaining Swiss cheese, cheddar cheese, spinach, cottage cheese, milk, eggs, and egg whites.

Whisk flour and baking powder in a small bowl. Add flour mixture to egg mixture and blend well. Pour egg mixture over ham and cheese. Bake for 45 minutes or until a knife inserted into the center of the quiche comes out clean.

NUTRITION PER SERVING | FAT: 9 GRAMS | CARBOHYDRATE: 17 GRAMS | PROTEIN: 24 GRAMS | TOTAL CALORIES: 245

VEGAN LENTIL SALAD

V

Lentils are powerhouses of nutrition. They're rich in folic acid and have a good amount of iron, potassium, protein, and thiamin, too. Plus, they cook quickly and taste delicious with just about anything. Delightfully spiked with garlic, this salad can be eaten right away or served as leftovers. In fact, it tastes better with time.

2 SERVINGS

1/2 cup lentils, rinsed and drained
1/2 yellow onion
1 garlic clove, crushed
1 bay leaf
1 red bell pepper, finely diced

1/2 red onion, chopped
2 tablespoons chopped parsley
2 teaspoons olive oil
2 teaspoons white wine vinegar

Bring a large pot of water to a boil over high heat. Add lentils, yellow onion, garlic, and bay leaf. Cook until lentils are just tender, 20 to 30 minutes. Drain; discard onion, garlic, and bay leaf.

Transfer lentils to a medium bowl and toss with bell peppers, red onions, parsley, oil, and vinegar. Season with salt and pepper. Cool before serving.

NUTRITION PER SERVING | FAT: 5 GRAMS | CARBOHYDRATE: 35 GRAMS | PROTEIN: 12 GRAMS | TOTAL CALORIES: 233

REFRESHING CUCUMBER SALAD WITH TUNA

The base of this salad is the Persian cucumber. Each is about 6 inches long, about half the size of a regular cucumber, and thin-skinned. You could also use English cucumbers, which are seedless and have a tasty thin skin as well. All cucumbers are a natural remedy for water retention and will help ease bloating.

4 SERVINGS

½ teaspoon grated lemon rind

3 tablespoons lemon juice

3 tablespoons olive oil

2 tablespoons red wine vinegar

2 teaspoons finely chopped fresh oregano

½ teaspoon kosher salt

¼ teaspoon black pepper

4 ounces canned tuna packed in water, drained

⅓ cup Kalamata olives, pitted and halved lengthwise

⅓ cup thinly sliced red onions

2 cups cherry tomatoes, halved

5–6 Persian cucumbers, halved lengthwise and cut into ½-inch-thick slices (about 3 cups)

4 ounces low-fat feta cheese, crumbled

In a large bowl, whisk together the lemon rind, lemon juice, oil, vinegar, oregano, salt, and pepper.

Add the tuna, olives, onions, tomatoes, and cucumbers; toss gently to combine. Sprinkle with feta cheese.

NUTRITION PER SERVING | **FAT: 16 GRAMS** | **CARBOHYDRATE: 11 GRAMS** | **PROTEIN: 12 GRAMS** | **TOTAL CALORIES: 236**

HOO-YA

5 THINGS THAT MAY SURPRISE YOU ABOUT CUCUMBERS

Did you know that cucumbers:

1. Contain most of the vitamins and many of the other nutrients you need every day, namely, vitamins C, B_1, B_2, B_3, B_5, and B_6, as well as folic acid, calcium, iron, magnesium, phosphorus, potassium, and zinc?

2. Can help prevent a hangover? Simply eat a few cucumber slices before going to bed. Cucumbers contain enough sugar, B vitamins, and electrolytes to replenish essential nutrients your body loses from overindulging.

3. Can relieve stress? Slice a whole cucumber and place the slices into a pot of boiling water. The steam will release a soothing, relaxing aroma.

4. Eliminate bad breath? Press a slice of cucumber to the roof of your mouth with your tongue for 30 seconds. The phytochemicals in the cucumber kill the bacteria in your mouth that cause bad breath.

5. Are really fruits, originating in India and cultivated as a nutritious food for more than three thousand years?

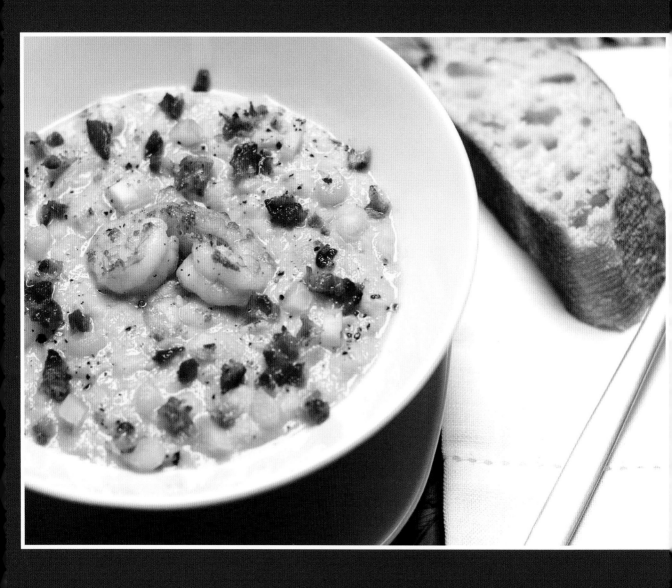

CORN CHOWDER WITH SHRIMP AND BACON

Think chowder, and seafood comes to mind. But back in the 1800s, New Englanders who moved west across the country couldn't find enough seafood or shellfish for their traditional chowders, so they substituted corn, which was more plentiful. And so, out of necessity was born a classic American dish—corn chowder. With my version, I decided to blend the best of both chowder worlds by adding shrimp.

4 SERVINGS

6 slices meaty bacon, chopped

1 cup chopped onions

1/2 cup chopped celery

1 teaspoon chopped fresh thyme

1 garlic clove, minced

4 cups corn kernels, fresh or canned

2 cups low-sodium, low-fat chicken broth

3/4 pound peeled and deveined medium shrimp

1/3 cup half-and-half

Heat a large pot over medium-high heat. Add bacon and cook until bacon begins to brown. Take out half the bacon and drain on paper towels.

To the bacon in the pan, add the onions, celery, thyme, and garlic and sauté for 2 minutes. Add the corn and cook for 2 minutes more. Add the broth, bring to a boil, then reduce heat and simmer 4 minutes.

Remove 2 cups of the corn mixture and whirl in a blender until smooth. Return the pureed corn mixture to pot. Stir in the shrimp and cook for 2 minutes, until shrimp is pink. Stir in half-and-half and season with salt and pepper. Crumble reserved bacon over the soup.

NUTRITION PER SERVING | FAT: 13 GRAMS | CARBOHYDRATE: 45 GRAMS | PROTEIN: 29 GRAMS | TOTAL CALORIES: 413

ZUCCHINI AND SALMON SALAD

I love salads, but sometimes I get bored with lettuce. This salad turns over a new leaf; it doesn't use lettuce at all, relying on zucchini as the tasty base for salmon, which is high in omega-3s.

4 SERVINGS

1 tablespoon olive oil

Four 2-ounce salmon fillets

3 large shallots, thinly sliced

4 zucchini, sliced in 1/4-inch rounds

11/2 teaspoons kosher salt

3 to 4 tablespoons lime juice

1 tablespoon brown sugar

1 tablespoon fish sauce

1 garlic clove, minced

1/4 teaspoon grated ginger

1/4 cup chopped cilantro

Heat a skillet over medium-high heat and add the oil. Cook the salmon 3–4 minutes on each side, until browned and cooked through; set aside. Add the shallots to the pan and cook for 3–5 minutes, until browned; set aside.

In a pot of boiling water, blanch the zucchini for 1 minute. Drain in a colander, sprinkle with a pinch of the kosher salt, and gently toss to coat; set aside to drain.

In a medium bowl, whisk 3 tablespoons lime juice, brown sugar, fish sauce, garlic, remaining salt, and ginger until sugar dissolves.

Add the zucchini and cilantro to the lime juice mixture and toss to coat; taste and add remaining 1 tablespoon lime juice if desired. Transfer to a shallow serving dish and top with the salmon and shallots. Drizzle remaining oil from the pan over salad.

NUTRITION PER SERVING | FAT: 11 GRAMS | CARBOHYDRATE: 17 GRAMS | PROTEIN: 14 GRAMS | TOTAL CALORIES: 223

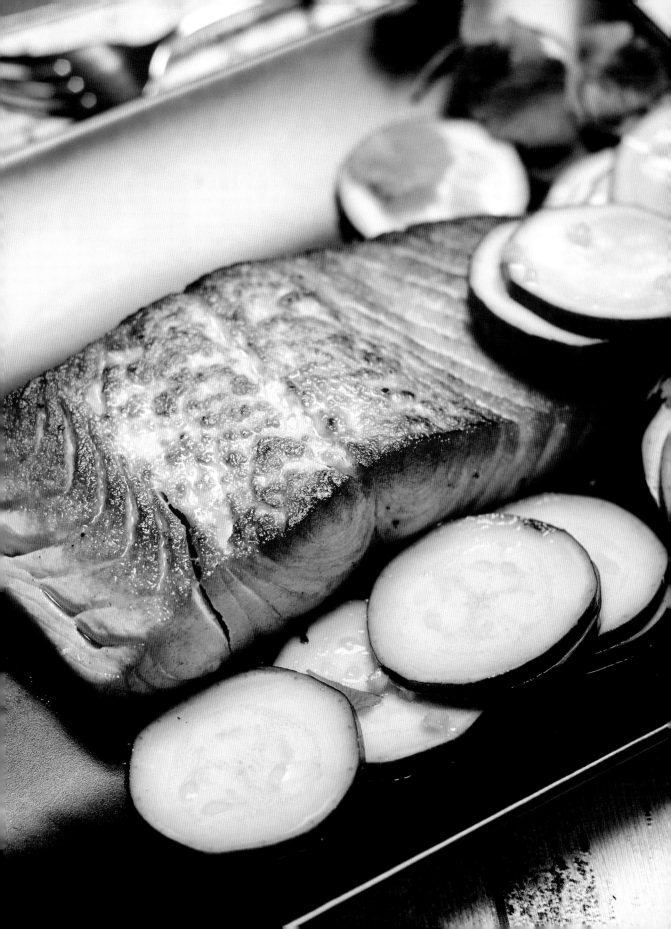

GRILLED SHRIMP AND SPINACH SALAD

Here's what I call a filling entrée salad. Shrimp is a great source of lean protein, and the spinach amps up fiber and phytonutrients. This recipe is ridiculously easy and amazingly yummy. With just a few ingredients, you can serve it up in no time.

6 SERVINGS

SHRIMP

2 pounds peeled and deveined large shrimp

2 teaspoons olive oil

1 teaspoon grated ginger

1/2 teaspoon ground cumin

2 garlic cloves, minced

DRESSING

2 tablespoons rice vinegar

2 tablespoons orange juice

11/2 tablespoons extra-virgin olive oil

1 tablespoon honey

1 tablespoon low-sodium soy sauce

1/2 teaspoon grated ginger

1/2 teaspoon salt

1/8 teaspoon crushed red pepper

SALAD

8 cups tightly packed baby spinach

2 cups thinly sliced shiitake mushroom caps

3/4 cup thinly sliced red onions

Toss the shrimp with oil, ginger, cumin, and garlic in a large bowl; season with salt and pepper. Thread about 5 shrimp onto each of six 8-inch skewers. Place skewers on a grill rack coated with cooking spray; grill 3 minutes, turning once, until the shrimp is pink and opaque.

Whisk the dressing ingredients together and set aside.

In a large bowl, combine the spinach, mushrooms, and onions. Add the dressing mixture and toss gently to coat. Serve with shrimp skewers.

NUTRITION PER SERVING | FAT: 9 GRAMS | CARBOHYDRATE: 9 GRAMS | PROTEIN: 41 GRAMS | TOTAL CALORIES: 281

SPICY SHRIMP COBB SALAD

This famous salad entrée is believed to have originated in the 1930s at Hollywood's Brown Derby restaurant, when it was created one late night from leftovers for the restaurant's owner, Robert Howard Cobb. Its usual components are egg, avocado, tomato, chicken or ham, bacon, and blue cheese, but I've changed up the recipe a bit.

4 SERVINGS

4 strips turkey bacon

1 pound peeled and deveined large shrimp

One 16-ounce package romaine salad

2 cups cherry tomatoes, halved

1 avocado, sliced

1 cup shredded carrots

1 cup frozen whole-kernel corn, thawed

1 teaspoon salt

21/2 tablespoons lemon juice

11/2 tablespoons olive oil

1/2 teaspoon paprika

1/4 teaspoon black pepper

1 teaspoon whole-grain brown mustard

Cook the bacon in a large skillet over medium heat until crisp. Drain on paper towels.

Coat the skillet with cooking spray and pan-fry the shrimp until golden brown.

Place the romaine, tomatoes, avocado, carrots, and corn in a large salad bowl.

In a small bowl, whisk together the salt, lemon juice, olive oil, paprika, pepper, and mustard. Pour the dressing over the salad and gently toss. Add shrimp. Crumble bacon over the top.

NUTRITION PER SERVING   FAT: 15 GRAMS   CARBOHYDRATE: 27 GRAMS   PROTEIN: 30 GRAMS   TOTAL CALORIES: 363

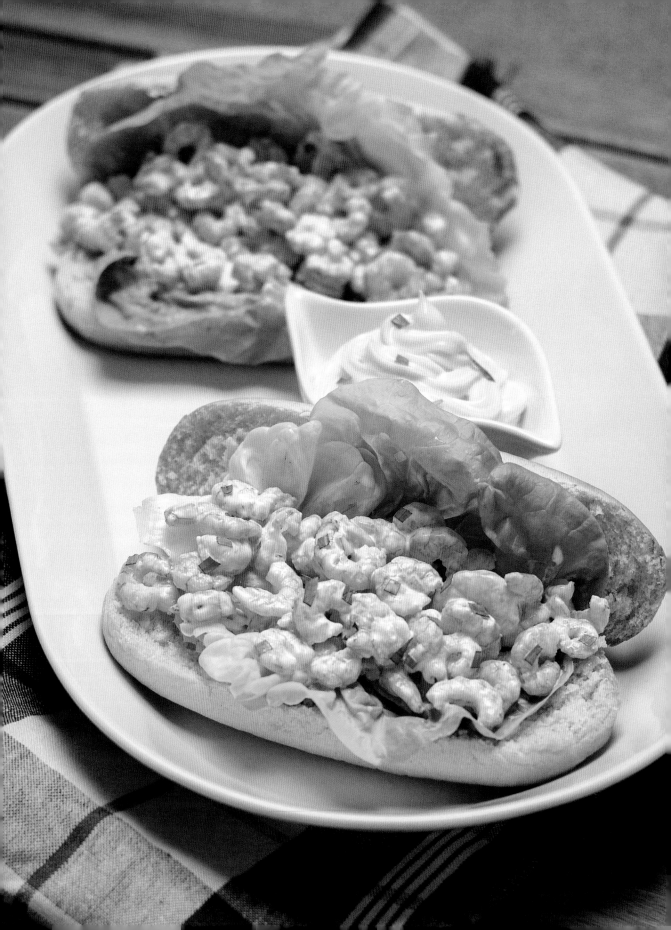

SHRIMP SALAD WRAPS

Here's a way to shed carbs and shed some weight at the same time. Fresh lettuce leaves serve as the wrap for a tasty shrimp filling. This crunchy handheld salad is light, tasty, and satisfying. If you want to make this a fast-fuel meal, simply place the shrimp salad wraps on baguettes, as shown in the photo.

4 SERVINGS

1 tablespoon lemon juice

1/3 cup low-fat mayonnaise

1 small shallot, minced

1 tablespoon finely chopped fresh tarragon

2 tablespoons chopped scallions

1 pound cooked shrimp, chopped

1/2 cup finely chopped celery

4 leaves Boston lettuce

Combine the lemon juice, mayonnaise, shallots, tarragon, and scallions in a large bowl. Add the shrimp and celery and toss gently. Season with salt and pepper.

Arrange 1 lettuce leaf on each plate. Divide the shrimp mixture evenly among lettuce leaves.

NUTRITION PER SERVING | FAT: 8 GRAMS | CARBOHYDRATE: 28 GRAMS | PROTEIN: 20 GRAMS | TOTAL CALORIES: 264

VIETNAMESE CHICKEN SALAD

There's a sandwich in Vietnamese cuisine called *banh mi* (BUN-mee) that features meat and is heavy on shredded cabbage, all encased in a crusty baguette. This recipe ditches the bread but serves up everything else, so you get all the flavor in this beloved Asian dish but none of the carbs. This chicken salad can be easily refrigerated and served as lunch several days in the same week.

6 SERVINGS

1 whole chicken

2 limes

1 small red onion, thinly sliced

1 teaspoon coarse Himalayan salt

1 teaspoon black pepper

1/2 head raw cabbage, thinly sliced

Vietnamese coriander (see sidebar)

1/2 bunch cilantro, leaves only, chopped

Place the chicken in a large pot, cover with water, and bring to a boil. Reduce heat and simmer the chicken, covered, 15–30 minutes, until cooked through. Remove the chicken and transfer it to a platter to cool. Shred the meat; discard bones and skin.

Squeeze the juice of 1 lime over the onions.

Combine the salt and pepper and sprinkle on the chicken, then toss the cabbage and chicken together. Add onions, coriander, and cilantro to the salad. Squeeze the juice of the second lime over the entire dish and toss all ingredients together.

HOO-YA

VIETNAMESE CORIANDER

Here is a wonderful culinary herb that looks like mint and smells like mint, but is not a member of the mint family. Used in Southeast Asian cooking, Vietnamese coriander is commonly eaten fresh in salads, in raw summer rolls, and in soups. You can find it in most Asian markets.

NUTRITION PER SERVING | FAT: 6 GRAMS | CARBOHYDRATE: 7 GRAMS | PROTEIN: 29 GRAMS | TOTAL CALORIES: 198

GARLIC CHICKEN BROCCOLINI SALAD

If you're a broccoli hater, try broccolini. It's a hybrid of broccoli and Chinese kale that tastes milder and sweeter than broccoli. It's still a cruciferous veggie, so it has all the nutritional and cancer-fighting benefits of broccoli.

4 SERVINGS

11/2 pounds broccolini

2 tablespoons olive oil

1 teaspoon butter

3 shallots, thinly sliced

2 large garlic cloves, minced

1/2 teaspoon crushed red pepper

1 cup shredded skinless, boneless rotisserie chicken breast

2 tablespoons shaved Parmesan cheese

1/2 cup chopped fresh chives

2 tablespoons pine nuts, toasted

Cut each piece of broccolini into thirds.

Heat the olive oil and butter in a large skillet or wok over medium-low heat. Add the shallots and cook, stirring, 4–5 minutes.

Add the garlic and crushed red pepper, and season with salt and pepper. Add the broccolini and cook until soft (but don't overcook it). Transfer the broccolini to a large bowl. Add the chicken to the bowl and toss. Sprinkle with cheese, chives, and pine nuts.

NUTRITION PER SERVING | FAT: 13 GRAMS | CARBOHYDRATE: 10 GRAMS | PROTEIN: 22 GRAMS | TOTAL CALORIES: 245

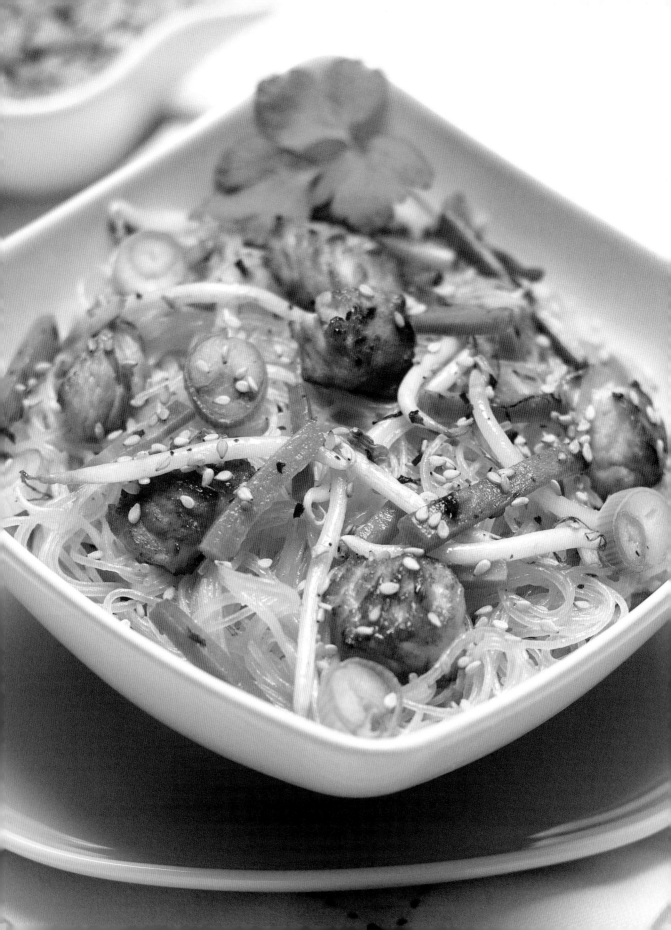

PAD THAI WITH KELP NOODLES

We all enjoy our little rituals, and one of mine involves eating pad Thai once a week. Traditional pad Thai is usually fried ("pad" means "stir-fry" in Thai), so it's not for the fitness-conscious person. But I can't go more than a week without some pad Thai, so I clearly had to find a way to create a more healthful version. My solution: using noodles made from sea kelp. They're available in Asian grocery stores and whole-foods stores. Kelp noodles have a mild flavor and are slightly crunchy. They are high in calcium and metabolism-boosting iodine. Plus they're super low in carbs, so this dish counts as a slow fuel.

2 SERVINGS

2 tablespoons almond butter

Crushed red pepper

4 tablespoons fish sauce

4 garlic cloves, minced

1/4 medium yellow onion, sliced

Juice of 1 lime (or 1 tablespoon white vinegar)

1 tablespoon olive oil

1/2 cup shredded carrot

3 ounces skinless, boneless chicken breast, diced

1 package kelp noodles, rinsed, drained, and towel-dried

2 cups fresh bean sprouts

Sriracha (optional)

1/2 cup chopped cilantro

1 scallion, sliced

1/4 cup roughly chopped peanuts

Sesame seeds

In a small bowl, mix the almond butter, crushed red pepper to taste, fish sauce, half the garlic, half the onions, and lime juice.

Heat a small skillet over medium heat. Add oil, the remaining onions, the remaining garlic, carrots, and chicken and sauté until chicken is cooked through. Add the kelp noodles and cook for 2 minutes. Transfer the mixture to a large bowl. Add bean sprouts to the chicken mixture. Add the sauce and mix well. Season with sriracha and additional fish sauce to taste.

Garnish with cilantro, scallions, peanuts, and sesame seeds.

NUTRITION PER SERVING | FAT: 20 GRAMS | CARBOHYDRATE: 12 GRAMS | PROTEIN: 20 GRAMS | TOTAL CALORIES: 308

TURKEY LETTUCE WRAPS

Deli food never goes out of style! In this recipe, I've tweaked a traditional deli turkey sandwich by dispensing with the bread and replacing it with lettuce leaves. Now, before you shout "Sacrilegious!" please taste it first. I'm sure you'll shout "Delicious!" instead.

2 SERVINGS

1 avocado
Juice of 1/2 lemon
Garlic powder
1/2 cup grape tomatoes, halved
1/4 bell pepper, diced

2 tablespoons chopped onions
1 tablespoon chopped cilantro
6 large lettuce leaves
6 deli turkey slices

Mash the avocado with a fork and add lemon juice. Add garlic powder to taste and season with salt and pepper. Mix in tomatoes, bell peppers, onions, and cilantro.

Place a lettuce leaf on a plate and top it with a turkey slice. Place a scoop of avocado mixture on the turkey, then wrap. Repeat with the rest of the lettuce leaves.

NUTRITION PER SERVING | FAT: 12 GRAMS | CARBOHYDRATE: 17 GRAMS | PROTEIN: 14 GRAMS | TOTAL CALORIES: 232

TACO LETTUCE BOATS

Lettuce is so versatile that it can even replace the fattening, salty taco in Mexican cuisine. The real taste of a taco is in the filling anyway. Once these Taco Lettuce Boats pass your lips, you won't miss that fried cornmeal taco one bit.

4 SERVINGS

1 tablespoon olive oil

1 pound ground turkey breast

1-ounce packaged taco seasoning

1 head romaine lettuce, leaves separated, washed, and dried

1 cup diced tomatoes

1/4 cup diced onions

1 cup shredded cheddar cheese

1/2 cup light sour cream

Salsa (optional)

Heat a large skillet over medium-high heat and add the oil. Add the ground turkey and brown. Add taco seasoning and water as directed on the packet and cook until the liquid disappears. Transfer to a bowl and set aside.

Place lettuce leaves on a platter and add turkey, tomatoes, onions, cheese, sour cream, and salsa (if using) to each one.

NUTRITION PER SERVING FAT: 14 GRAMS CARBOHYDRATE: 9 GRAMS PROTEIN: 36 GRAMS TOTAL CALORIES: 306

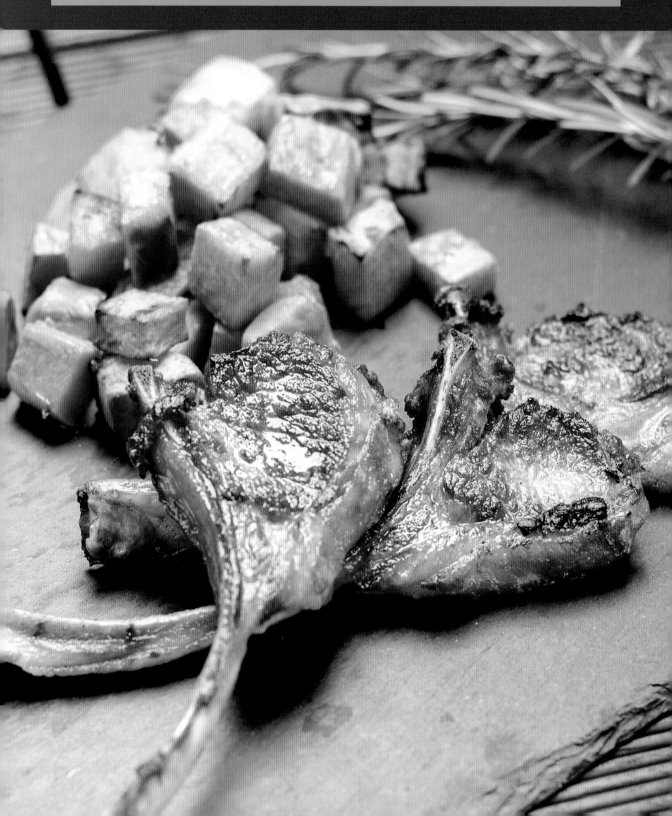

GRILLED ROSEMARY LAMB CHOPS

Did I hear someone say "grilled"? I love to grill pretty much any time of the year, and this recipe just shouts out "Grill me!" It takes about two seconds to whip up the marinade. The touch of sriracha makes for some tangy chops.

4 SERVINGS

1 tablespoon olive oil

1 tablespoon Himalayan salt

1 tablespoon black pepper

1 bunch fresh rosemary, leaves only, chopped

1 tablespoon sriracha

4 lamb chops

4 large carrots, peeled

Preheat oven to 350 degrees.

Combine the olive oil, salt, pepper, rosemary, and sriracha in a small bowl and mix well. Pour the mixture over the lamb chops, massage a bit into the meat, and then let the chops sit, covered, in the refrigerator 30–45 minutes.

Coat a baking sheet with cooking spray.

Cut the carrots into 1/2 inch rounds or cubes. Place them on the baking sheet and bake about 30 minutes, or until the carrots are soft.

Grill the lamb chops for about 7 minutes on each side, until done to your liking, and serve with the carrots.

NUTRITION PER SERVING | FAT: 11 GRAMS | CARBOHYDRATE: 6 GRAMS | PROTEIN: 23 GRAMS | TOTAL CALORIES: 217

ASIAN GINGER CHICKEN

Wake up your chicken with ginger, garlic, soy sauce, and sesame oil—a decidedly Asian flair.

2 SERVINGS

1 small carrot, julienned

1 small red bell pepper, julienned

1/4 cup sliced onions

1 cup shredded skinless, boneless rotisserie chicken breast

2 cups kelp noodles, rinsed, drained, and towel-dried

3 tablespoons almond butter

1 teaspoon miso (see sidebar)

1 tablespoon sesame oil

1 tablespoon ginger, grated

1 garlic clove, minced

1 tablespoon apple cider vinegar

1 scallion, sliced

1/2 cup chopped cilantro

Combine the carrots, peppers, onions, chicken, and kelp noodles in a bowl; set aside.

In a food processor, combine almond butter, miso, sesame oil, ginger, garlic, vinegar, and 1/2 cup water until smooth. Season with salt and pepper.

Pour sauce over noodle mixture and toss. Garnish with scallions and cilantro.

NUTRITION PER SERVING | FAT: 18 GRAMS | CARBOHYDRATE: 10 GRAMS | PROTEIN: 22 GRAMS | TOTAL CALORIES: 290

HOO-YA

MISO

An integral component of Japanese cuisine, miso (MEE-soh) is a thick, salty paste of fermented soybeans and grains with the consistency of peanut butter.

Depending on the recipe, miso is a flavor enhancer, curing agent, sauce thickener, fat substitute, or culinary cure-all. Some cooks use it liberally in place of oil in vinaigrettes and marinades.

One downside is that it is fairly high in sodium, so you've got to use small amounts of it. If you're concerned about sodium, talk to your physician.

Miso is also believed to have significant nutritional and medicinal properties. Like yogurt, it contains live cultures, including lactobacillus, which is believed to promote digestion and assimilation of nutrients during digestion. Miso is loaded with antioxidants and contains protein in the form of easy-to-digest amino acids, as well as minerals and vitamins, particularly vitamin B_{12} (making it great for vegetarians, since B_{12} is found mostly in meat). Clearly, there's a lot going for miso.

CHICKEN ZOODLES CHOW MEIN

Take away any of the fancy gadgets in my kitchen—but please don't take away my spiralizer. This handy little device works like a pencil sharpener and turns vegetables such as yellow squash or zucchini into low-carb noodles that can take the place of pasta in any recipe.

4 SERVINGS

1 pound ground chicken breast

1 teaspoon grated ginger

1 teaspoon fish sauce

1 teaspoon low-sodium soy sauce

6 medium yellow squash

2 teaspoons salt

2 tablespoons olive oil

3 garlic cloves, minced

1 tablespoon sriracha (optional)

3/4 cup thinly sliced yellow onions

1/2 cup shredded carrots

1 tablespoon sesame oil

1 tablespoon sesame seeds

1 scallion, chopped

1/2 cup chopped cilantro

In a bowl, combine the chicken, ginger, fish sauce, and soy sauce; season with salt and pepper. Cover and marinate for an hour in the refrigerator.

Use a spiralizer to turn the squash into "zoodles" and place in a large bowl. Add the salt and toss lightly. Set aside at room temperature for 30 minutes. Drain liquid. Spread zoodles on a large clean towel. Place in the refrigerator for 1 hour uncovered to dehydrate.

Heat a large pan or wok on medium-high heat and add 1 tablespoon olive oil and the garlic. Once the garlic is golden, add the chicken mixture and sriracha. Cook 3–5 minutes, until the chicken is cooked through; transfer to a plate. In the same pan, heat the other tablespoon of olive oil and cook the onions and carrots until the carrots are tender; transfer to the plate with the chicken.

In the same pan, heat the sesame oil. Blot the zoodles with a paper towel and add to pan. Stir-fry for 5 minutes or until soft. Add the chicken and onion mixture to the pan and heat through. Season with salt and pepper. Garnish with sesame seeds, scallions, and cilantro.

NUTRITION PER SERVING | FAT: 14 GRAMS | CARBOHYDRATE: 19 GRAMS | PROTEIN: 31 GRAMS | TOTAL CALORIES: 326

HOO-YA

OTHER WAYS TO DRY YOUR ZOODLES

Zucchini and yellow squash are very moist vegetables. If you turn them into zoodles with your spiralizer and you want to eat them raw, you should make sure to dry them.

There are two ways to dry zoodles. One is to "sweat" them. Sprinkle zoodles generously with salt, and toss to coat well. Place the zoodles on a cookie sheet lined with paper towels. "Sweat" the zoodles in the oven on low heat (200 degrees) for 30 minutes, until the paper towels have absorbed most of the moisture. Wrap the paper towels around the zoodles and squeeze to extract any remaining liquid.

The other way is to place the zoodles in a colander, salt generously, toss to coat well, and let them sit for about twenty minutes. Then wrap the zoodles in a paper towel and gently squeeze them to extract as much moisture (and salt) as possible. Spread them on a towel and let them sit in the refrigerator for 30 minutes.

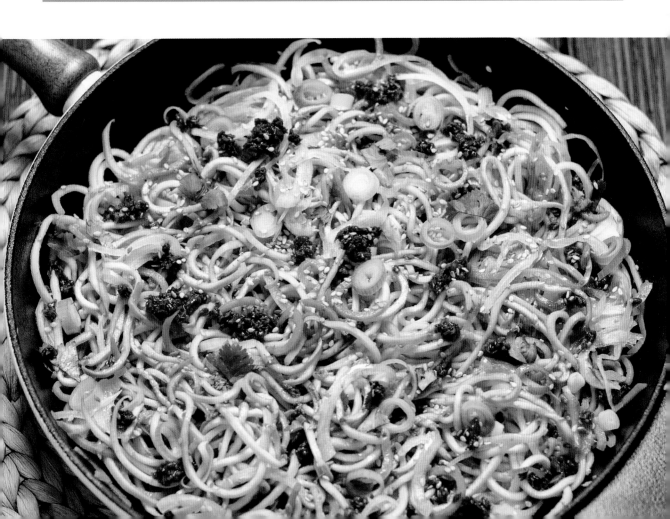

BLACKENED GROUPER AND SNAP PEAS

Grouper is one of the meatiest, moistest white fish you can eat. When you blacken it, as shown here, expect every bite to explode with flavor.

4 SERVINGS

Four 4-ounce grouper fillets

3 tablespoons olive oil

1 teaspoon dried thyme

1 teaspoon paprika

1 teaspoon black pepper

1/2 teaspoon salt

1/4 teaspoon five-spice powder

3 cups sugar snap peas

2 garlic cloves, minced

Rinse the fish and pat dry with a paper towel. Mix 1 tablespoon oil, the thyme, paprika, pepper, salt, and five-spice powder in a small bowl. Spread the mixture over the fish and let marinate for about 30 minutes.

Wash the snap peas and pat dry. Preheat a skillet over high heat and add 1 tablespoon oil. Add snap peas and stir-fry 3 minutes. Add the garlic and stir-fry for another 3 minutes. Season with salt and pepper.

Heat another pan over medium heat and add the last tablespoon of olive oil. Pan-fry the fish 5–7 minutes on each side, until golden brown. Serve with snap peas.

NUTRITION PER SERVING   FAT: 12 GRAMS   CARBOHYDRATE: 5 GRAMS   PROTEIN: 22 GRAMS   TOTAL CALORIES: 216

TANDOORI CHICKEN AND CUCUMBER SALAD

Tandoori chicken is one of my favorite Indian dishes. It is named for the tandoor, a clay oven fired with hot coals, in which the chicken is cooked. You don't have to have a special oven to create a perfectly respectable version, though! My version uses all of the key ingredients to capture the exotic flavor and aroma of the traditional Indian dish. And as they'd do in India (or an Indian restaurant), I pair it with a light, refreshing cucumber salad.

4 SERVINGS

2 cups plain whole-milk yogurt

11/2 tablespoons grated ginger

11/2 tablespoons minced garlic

2 teaspoons ground coriander

2 teaspoons paprika

1/2 teaspoon cayenne

3 tablespoons lime juice

11/2 pounds skinless, boneless chicken breast

1 English cucumber, diced

1/2 cup cherry tomatoes, halved

1/4 cup diced onions

1 tablespoon olive oil

1/4 cup chopped cilantro

In a large bowl, combine the yogurt, ginger, garlic, coriander, paprika, cayenne, and 1 tablespoon lime juice. Add chicken, turn to coat, and marinate for 1 hour or longer in refrigerator.

Preheat oven to 400 degrees. Coat a baking dish with cooking spray.

In a large bowl, toss the cucumbers, tomatoes, onions, olive oil, and 2 tablespoons lime juice. Season with salt and pepper and set aside.

Remove the chicken from the marinade and place in the baking dish. Bake 10–20 minutes, turning once, until nearly done. Spread remaining marinade on top and bake another 5–10 minutes, until cooked through. Serve with cucumber salad and garnish with cilantro.

NUTRITION PER SERVING | **FAT: 12 GRAMS** | **CARBOHYDRATE: 13 GRAMS** | **PROTEIN: 43 GRAMS** | **TOTAL CALORIES: 333**

TILAPIA AND DILL IN PARCHMENT

Delicate fish like tilapia is easily baked *en papillote* (in parchment paper). The parchment is folded tightly and baked, thus steaming the fish and veggies and locking in the intermingling flavors. You can use this cooking method with any type of fish, and it's guaranteed to create a tender, delicious seafood meal. (If you want to turn this dish into a fast fuel, serve it with a side of wild rice.)

4 SERVINGS

Four 3-ounce tilapia fillets
1 cup chopped tomatoes
1/2 cup chopped onions
3 garlic cloves, minced
3/4 cup chopped fresh dill

4 teaspoons lemon juice
2 tablespoons olive oil
1 cup white wine
11/2 teaspoons capers

Preheat oven to 350 degrees.

In a large bowl, toss the fish with the remaining ingredients. Season with salt and pepper.

Prepare 4 sheets of parchment paper (about 12 inches square each) by folding each sheet in half and placing tilapia mixture on one side of the fold of each sheet. Roll up the edges of the paper, making a crescent moon, and tuck the ends under.

Place parchment packets on a baking sheet and bake 15–20 minutes, until the tilapia is cooked through.

NUTRITION PER SERVING FAT: 9 GRAMS CARBOHYDRATE: 16 GRAMS PROTEIN: 26 GRAMS TOTAL CALORIES: 249

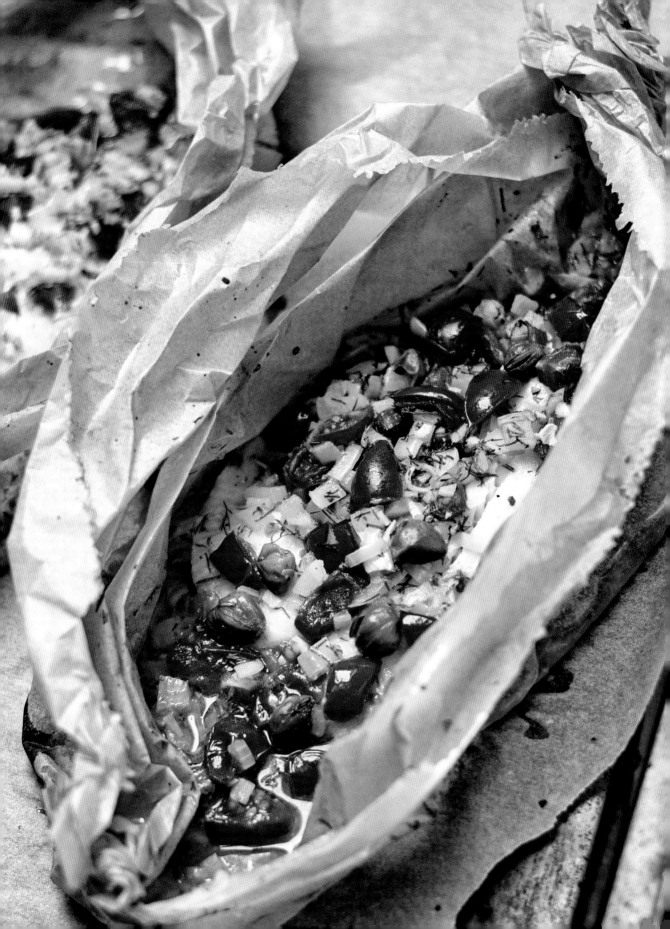

CHICKEN PARMESAN WITH SPAGHETTI SQUASH

By definition, traditional chicken Parmesan is a fat and carb bomb. That's because the recipe usually calls for breaded and fried chicken smothered in an oil-heavy sauce and topped with piles of cheese. And it's usually served with a boatload of pasta to boot! However, there is a way to enjoy this classic dish without all the fattening calories. This recipe shows you how.

2 SERVINGS

1 spaghetti squash
2 skinless, boneless chicken breasts
1 teaspoon dried oregano
1 tablespoon minced garlic

1 cup low-sugar or low-carbohydrate pasta sauce
1 cup shredded fat-free mozzarella cheese
1/2 cup chopped parsley

Preheat oven to 375 degrees.

Poke holes in the squash with a knife and microwave the squash 3–5 minutes, until it begins to soften somewhat. Cut the squash in half lengthwise and scoop out the seeds with a spoon. Season with salt and pepper.

Coat a baking sheet with cooking spray and place squash cut side down. Bake for 30 minutes, until a fork can go through the middle of squash and the flesh is soft.

Sprinkle the chicken with the oregano and garlic, and season with salt and pepper. Coat a skillet with cooking spray and heat over medium-high heat. Brown chicken on both sides and cook until done. Cut chicken into small pieces.

Remove the squash from the oven and flip over. Use a fork and rake the inside to create spaghetti-like strands. To each squash half add half the chicken and 1/2 cup spaghetti sauce. Top with 1/2 cup mozzarella. Bake the filled squash 10–15 minutes, until the cheese is melted. Garnish with parsley.

NUTRITION PER SERVING | FAT: 5 GRAMS | CARBOHYDRATE: 43 GRAMS | PROTEIN: 50 GRAMS | TOTAL CALORIES: 417

PESTO CHICKEN BAKE

A great way to flavor otherwise boring chicken breasts is to spread each one with pesto and top with tomatoes and shredded cheese. So easy, so fast, and so delicious!

4 SERVINGS

2 skinless, boneless chicken breasts

4 tablespoons store-bought pesto

1 large tomato, cut into 4 slices

1 cup shredded reduced-fat mozzarella cheese

1 handful chopped fresh basil

3 cups torn lettuce

1 cup cherry tomatoes

1/2 cup sliced cucumber

1/4 cup Italian dressing

Preheat oven to 400 degrees. Coat a baking dish with cooking spray.

Cut chicken breasts in half lengthwise, season with salt and pepper, and place in baking dish. Spread 1 tablespoon pesto on top of each piece of chicken. Top each with a tomato slice and a quarter of the cheese. Bake chicken for 30 minutes or until cooked through. Garnish with basil.

In a large bowl, toss the lettuce, cherry tomatoes, and cucumber with the dressing. Serve alongside the chicken.

NUTRITION PER SERVING | **FAT: 11 GRAMS** | CARBOHYDRATE: 8 GRAMS | **PROTEIN: 21 GRAMS** | **TOTAL CALORIES: 215**

BALSAMIC CHICKEN

Balsamic vinegar is a versatile pantry staple to have on hand. You can use it in marinades and sauces, or you can drizzle it over fruit, vegetables, meats, seafood, or chicken. In this recipe, you'll take this dark vinegar to another taste level by reducing it, along with other ingredients, to a nice syrupy consistency that gives the chicken a tasty glaze.

4 SERVINGS

1 tablespoon olive oil

2 cups 2-inch pieces green beans

1 cup sliced mushrooms

1 cup 2-inch pieces asparagus

11/2 pounds skinless, boneless chicken breast, cut into 8 pieces

1/4 cup light Italian dressing

1 tablespoon agave syrup

3 tablespoons balsamic vinegar

1 cup grape tomatoes

Heat a large pan over medium-high heat. Add the oil, green beans, mushrooms, and asparagus. Cook until the green beans are tender. Transfer to a large plate.

Add the chicken to the pan and season with salt and pepper. Cook chicken 3–5 minutes on each side, until done. Remove chicken.

In the same pan, combine Italian dressing, agave, and vinegar and stir well. Add the vegetable mixture, chicken, and tomatoes. Cook, stirring, another 3–5 minutes. Transfer to plates and drizzle with remaining sauce from the pan.

NUTRITION PER SERVING | FAT: 9 GRAMS | CARBOHYDRATE: 22 GRAMS | PROTEIN: 41 GRAMS | TOTAL CALORIES: 333

HERBED CHICKEN BREASTS

The dish has a light touch of Italian influence in its use of garlic, basil, and oregano. Spiced with garlic, the green beans make the perfect side dish.

6 SERVINGS

6 skinless, boneless chicken breasts

3 tablespoons olive oil

1/2 cup chopped fresh basil

2 tablespoons finely chopped fresh oregano

4 garlic cloves, minced

1 tablespoon finely chopped fresh thyme

1 teaspoon cayenne

2 pounds string beans

Place one chicken breast in a plastic bag or between two pieces of plastic wrap and flatten with a meat pounder or rolling pin until chicken is about 1/2 inch thick. Repeat with the other five breasts.

In a large bowl, whisk together 2 tablespoons oil, the basil, oregano, half the garlic, thyme, and cayenne; season with salt and pepper. Add the chicken and coat evenly. Cover the chicken and place it in the refrigerator for at least 1 hour.

Preheat oven to 400 degrees.

Arrange the chicken in a roasting pan and roast until done, about 30 minutes. Transfer to a platter.

Heat a skillet over medium-high heat. Add the remaining 1 tablespoon oil and the remaining garlic and cook until garlic is golden. Add string beans and cook 3–5 minutes, until tender. Season with salt and pepper. Serve with the chicken.

NUTRITION PER SERVING | FAT: 12 GRAMS | CARBOHYDRATE: 12 GRAMS | PROTEIN: 25 GRAMS | TOTAL CALORIES: 256

TRI-TIP AND BROCCOLINI

Tri-tip is a delicious, boneless cut of beef recognizable for its triangular shape. Considered a lower-fat cut, it has just enough internal fat to make it tender and tasty. My marinade makes it extra delicious!

4 SERVINGS

3 tablespoons brown mustard

1 tablespoon salt

1 tablespoon black pepper

1 tablespoon sriracha

4 garlic cloves, minced

16 ounces tri-tip, cut into 4 pieces

1 tablespoon olive oil

3 cups 1-inch pieces broccolini

2 cups sliced button mushrooms

Combine the mustard, salt, pepper, sriracha, and 2 garlic cloves. Cover the tri-tip with the mixture and marinate 45 minutes in the refrigerator.

Preheat a skillet or wok over high heat. Add the oil, remaining 2 garlic cloves, and broccolini and sauté 3–5 minutes. Add the mushrooms and cook 2 minutes more. Season with salt and pepper.

Preheat a grill to medium-high and grill meat 5–7 minutes each side, until done to your liking. Serve the meat with the vegetables.

NUTRITION PER SERVING FAT: 10 GRAMS CARBOHYDRATE: 10 GRAMS PROTEIN: 28 GRAMS TOTAL CALORIES: 242

CAULIFLOWER SKILLET

Here's a wonderful dish that serves double duty as either an entrée or, without the egg on top, a side dish. It's accented by bacon, something I could eat on everything—well, except ice cream.

2 SERVINGS

1 tablespoon olive oil

2 garlic cloves, minced

1/2 cup diced onions

1 pound cauliflower florets, chopped

2 bacon slices, cooked and crumbled

1/4 teaspoon paprika

2 teaspoon lemon juice

1/4 cup chopped tomatoes

1 tablespoon chopped parsley

2 large eggs

In a large skillet, heat oil over medium-high heat. Add the garlic and onions and cook until tender. Add the cauliflower and bacon and cook for 1 minute. Add 3 tablespoons water and the paprika, season with salt and pepper, and cook until the cauliflower is tender. Add the lemon juice, tomatoes, and parsley. Stir and transfer to a plate.

Coat a skillet with cooking spray and heat over medium-high heat. Crack the eggs into the skillet and cook until the egg whites are set. Slide one fried egg on top of each plate of cauliflower.

NUTRITION PER SERVING   FAT: 9 GRAMS   CARBOHYDRATE: 19 GRAMS   PROTEIN: 9 GRAMS   TOTAL CALORIES: 193

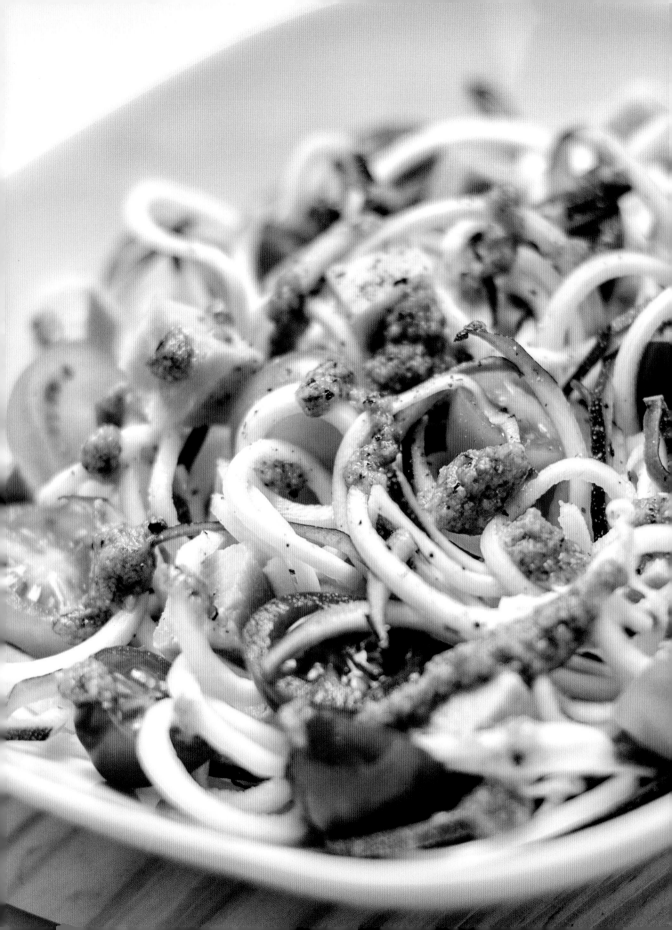

HAM PESTO ZOODLES

Ham goes Italian here, and it's fantastic. The sauce is a traditional pesto, made with basil, that accents the ham beautifully. And who needs noodles when you can make zoodles?

4 SERVINGS

1 cup tightly packed fresh basil

2 garlic cloves, minced

1/4 cup grated Parmesan cheese

3 tablespoons olive oil

5–6 medium zucchini

1 cup diced ham

1 cup chopped tomatoes

In a food processor, combine the basil, garlic, and Parmesan cheese and process. With the motor running, slowly add the oil until a smooth paste forms. Season with salt and pepper.

Spiralize the zucchini into a large bowl. Toss the zucchini with the ham, pesto, and tomatoes.

NUTRITION PER SERVING   FAT: 16 GRAMS   CARBOHYDRATE: 21 GRAMS   PROTEIN: 35 GRAMS   TOTAL CALORIES: 368

MUSHROOMS, TOFU, AND BABY BOK CHOY

With its mild cabbage taste, bok choy is a small green often used in Asian dishes as a bed for tofu or seafood. This dish is a great option for vegetarians and vegans— anyone, really—who wants to enjoy a meatless main course brimming with flavor.

4 SERVINGS

2 tablespoons olive oil

1 tablespoon grated ginger

1 cup chopped red onions

3 garlic cloves, minced

3 small carrots, peeled and sliced on an angle

6 baby bok choy, bottom trimmed and cut into halves

11/2 cups button mushrooms, halved

One 14-ounce package firm tofu, cut into small cubes

2 tablespoons soy sauce

1 teaspoon black pepper

1/2 cup thinly sliced scallions

Heat a skillet or wok over medium-high heat. Add the oil, ginger, onions, garlic, carrots, and bok choy and stir-fry 5 minutes. Add the mushrooms, tofu, soy sauce, and pepper and toss gently. Cook for 3–5 minutes more, until heated through. Garnish with scallions.

NUTRITION PER SERVING | FAT: 13 GRAMS | CARBOHYDRATE: 18 GRAMS | PROTEIN: 21 GRAMS | TOTAL CALORIES: 273

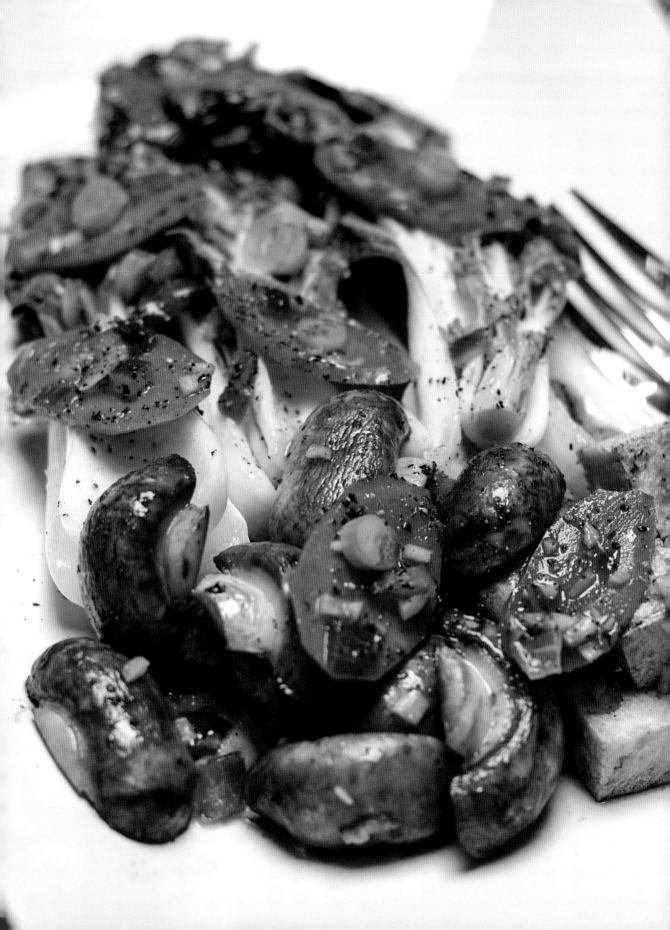

FILET MIGNON SKEWERS

Unless you're a strict vegan, you're bound to crave a meat-based meal from time to time. Here's one you'll love. It's a twist on the steakhouse classic, served with a variety of super-healthful, super-tasty veggies.

6 SERVINGS

11/2 pounds lean filet mignon, cut into big cubes

1 tablespoon kosher salt (or Himalayan salt if you have it)

1 tablespoon black pepper

1 large red onion, cut into large chunks

3 large portobello mushrooms, cut into large chunks

1 large green bell pepper, cut into large chunks

2 large zucchini, cut into thick slices

2 tablespoons olive oil

Preheat the grill to medium-high. Season filet mignon with the salt and pepper and allow to sit for 30 minutes.

If you're using wooden skewers, make sure you soak them in water for a few hours before using. If you're using metal skewers, coat them with cooking spray. Thread vegetables and meat onto the skewers, alternating one chunk of meat and one chunk of vegetable. Brush the skewered food with oil. Grill the skewers 2–3 minutes on each side, until done to your liking.

NUTRITION PER SERVING | FAT: 11 GRAMS | CARBOHYDRATE: 9 GRAMS | PROTEIN: 29 GRAMS | TOTAL CALORIES: 251

VEGAN SLOW COOKER CHILI

V

If you want to go meatless some evening, here's your go-to recipe. The imitation ground meat and kidney beans serve up all the protein you need. Just put the main ingredients in the slow cooker, and in several hours you have a robustly flavored, nutritious dinner. Save the leftovers for another meal.

8 SERVINGS

1 package imitation ground meat

1 package chili seasoning

One 15-ounce can kidney beans

Two 15-ounce cans diced tomatoes and green chiles

1 cup chopped onions

1 tablespoon minced garlic

1 green bell pepper, chopped

One 28-ounce can crushed tomatoes

1/2 teaspoon dried oregano

1/2 cup chopped cilantro

Combine all ingredients except cilantro in a slow cooker and season with salt and pepper. Cook on high for 4 hours. Garnish with cilantro.

NUTRITION PER SERVING | FAT: 3 GRAMS | CARBOHYDRATE: 30 GRAMS | PROTEIN: 14 GRAMS | TOTAL CALORIES: 257

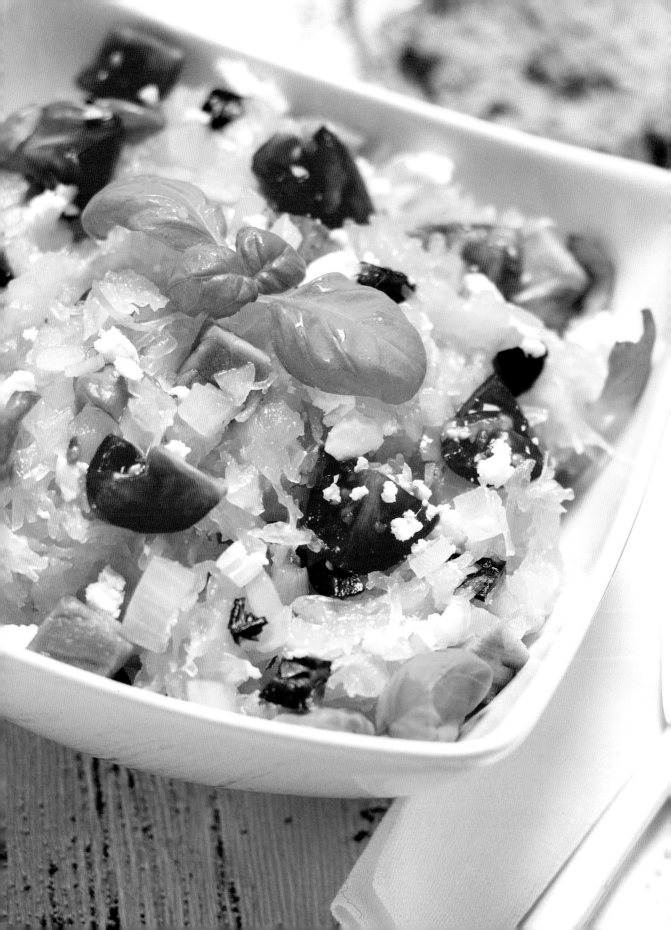

SPAGHETTI SQUASH WITH MEDITERRANEAN SCRAMBLE

Spaghetti squash has become the go-to substitute when you don't want high-carb pasta with your Italian dish. In this recipe, I've taken spaghetti sauce to a different part of the Mediterranean and to a different cuisine—Greek, by adding black olives and feta cheese to the dish.

2 SERVINGS

1 spaghetti squash, halved lengthwise and seeded

1 tablespoon olive oil

1 garlic clove, minced

1 cup diced hamsteak

1 cup chopped onions

11/2 cups chopped tomatoes

2/4 cup crumbled low-fat feta cheese

3 tablespoons chopped black olives

3 tablespoons chopped fresh basil

1/2 baguette, sliced 1 inch thick

Preheat oven to 350 degrees.

Coat a baking sheet with cooking spray and place squash cut side down. Bake for 30 minutes, until a fork can go through the middle of the squash and the flesh is soft.

Heat a large skillet over medium-high heat. Add oil, garlic, ham, and onions and cook until onions are soft. Add the tomatoes and cook until warmed through.

Scoop the spaghetti-like pulp from the squash into a large bowl and toss with the onion mixture, feta cheese, olives, and basil. Season with salt and pepper. Serve warm with sliced baguette.

NUTRITION PER SERVING | FAT: 16 GRAMS | CARBOHYDRATE: 33 GRAMS | FAT: 32 GRAMS | TOTAL CALORIES: 404

CAULIFLOWER CASSEROLE

Here's a veggie-packed recipe you could serve for breakfast, lunch, or dinner, or as a side dish. For vegetarians who eat eggs and dairy, it's the perfect entrée, too.

5 SERVINGS

1 large head cauliflower, core removed, cut into florets

1 red bell pepper, chopped

¾ cup shredded reduced-fat sharp cheddar cheese

¾ cup shredded Swiss cheese

10 large eggs, lightly beaten

½ cup chopped onions

1 cup low-fat milk

½ teaspoon garlic powder

½ teaspoon onion powder

½ cup chopped fresh dill

Preheat oven to 350 degrees. Coat a baking dish with cooking spray.

Add the cauliflower florets and bell peppers to a large pan and cover with 2 inches of water. Cover pan and steam over medium heat 5–7 minutes, until cauliflower is tender. Drain vegetables and transfer to the baking dish.

Set aside some of the cheese for a topping. In a bowl, combine the eggs, onions, milk, the remaining cheese, garlic powder, and onion powder. Pour the egg mixture over the cauliflower, top with the reserved cheese, and bake for 40 minutes, until cheese is golden brown. Garnish with dill.

NUTRITION PER SERVING | **FAT: 18 GRAMS** | **CARBOHYDRATE: 18 GRAMS** | **PROTEIN: 26 GRAMS** | **TOTAL CALORIES: 338**

CRABMEAT-STUFFED AVOCADO

For a slow-fuel snack, this one packs a lot of nutritional power: protein from crab-meat, antioxidants from the veggies, and good fat from the avocado. You can also enjoy this dish as a lunch; simply eat two avocado halves instead of just one.

6 SERVINGS

6 ounces crabmeat

2 tablespoons diced red bell peppers

2 tablespoons diced red onions

2 tablespoons diced celery

1 tablespoon chopped cilantro

11/2 tablespoons low-fat mayonnaise

Juice of 1 lime (optional)

1/8 teaspoon cayenne

3 avocados, halved and pitted

Mix together all the ingredients except the avocados; season with salt and pepper. Divide the crabmeat mixture evenly among the avocado halves.

NUTRITION PER SERVING | FAT: 16 GRAMS | CARBOHYDRATE: 10 GRAMS | PROTEIN: 21 GRAMS | TOTAL CALORIES: 268

STUFFED EGGS

Ah, stuffed eggs. Everyone's favorite at picnics and family gatherings. There are countless ways to stuff eggs, and here I've crammed them with lots of vegetables, accented by high-protein tuna.

5 SERVINGS

10 large eggs

Two 5-ounce cans tuna packed in water, drained

1/2 teaspoon brown mustard

1/4 cup chopped dill pickle

1 tablespoon low-fat mayonnaise

2 teaspoons lemon juice

6 crackers, crumbled

1 scallion, chopped

Paprika

2 cups baby carrots

6 celery stalks, cut into 3-inch pieces

1 cucumber, sliced

Boil a pot of water over medium-high heat. Cook eggs for 10 minutes. Drain, then place the eggs into cold water with ice cubes to stop the cooking; let sit 5 minutes. Peel eggs and cut in half; remove yolks and set whites aside.

In a bowl, mash the yolks and add the tuna, mustard, pickle, mayonnaise, lemon juice, and cracker crumbs; season with salt and pepper. Divide the tuna mixture among the egg whites. Garnish with scallions and paprika. Serve with a side of carrots, celery sticks, and sliced cucumbers.

NUTRITION PER SERVING | FAT: 11 GRAMS | CARBOHYDRATE: 10 GRAMS | PROTEIN: 21 GRAMS | TOTAL CALORIES: 223

CUCUMBER TUNA BOATS

There are as many ways to slice a cucumber as there are recipes. One of the best ways is lengthwise, with the seeds scooped out to make a boat that can be filled with a light, delicious tuna salad, as this recipe shows.

4 SERVINGS

2 English cucumbers

1/2 teaspoon Dijon mustard

1 tablespoon olive oil

1/4 cup plain low-fat yogurt

1/4 cup chopped fresh dill

2 tablespoons low-fat mayonnaise

2 scallions, sliced

1 stalk celery, thinly sliced

11/2 dill pickles, finely chopped

Two 5-ounce cans chunk light tuna packed in water, drained

Halve the cucumbers lengthwise; use a spoon to scoop out the seeds to make a boat shape.

Whisk together the mustard and oil in a medium bowl. Add the yogurt, dill, mayonnaise, scallions, celery, and pickles; season with salt and pepper. Stir in the drained tuna.

Fill each cucumber half with the tuna salad and serve.

NUTRITION PER SERVING FAT: 7 GRAMS CARBOHYDRATE: 4 GRAMS PROTEIN: 19 GRAMS TOTAL CALORIES: 155

Chapter 5

Smoothies and Juices

FUELING SMOOTHIES AND JUICES

SMOOTHIES

I'm a fan of smoothies as a snack in between meals. To me, whipping up a smoothie is how cooking should be: quick and easy, with very little cleanup. Toss a bunch of healthful stuff in the blender, punch a button, and seconds later you're in business. Also, studies have consistently proven that drinking a protein shake immediately after a workout creates a hormonal environment in the body that is conducive to muscle repair and growth.

My smoothies are made with non-dairy milk (almond, coconut, or rice milk) and a plant-based protein powder. These powders are typically formulated with brown rice, pea, hemp, or quinoa protein. (If you'd rather not go with plant-based protein powders, I suggest you try a whey protein powder. Whey is an ingredient with some terrific fat-burning and muscle-building perks.) To this base you can add fresh fruit or green leafy vegetables such as spinach or kale, plus your daily allotment of flax-seed, olive, or coconut oil.

FUELING JUICING

If you have trouble eating all your veggies or you just don't really like the taste of most of them, juicing may be a great solution for you. Juicing is an easy way to effectively mainline most of the nutrition of vegetables (though not the fiber)—an instant surge of vitamins and minerals. Fresh juices contain digestive enzymes that work to scrub away toxins in your digestive tract, revitalizing your entire system. They're also loaded with phytochemicals, natural substances in plants that promote good health and defend the body against diseases.

Another reason I promote juicing is that it helps fight food cravings. If you've tried to lose weight in the past but felt hungry for sweets and other foods all the time, it could be because you lacked some essential vitamins and minerals. Juicing helps replenish those elements and satisfy a sweet tooth. The net effect is that you may eat less of the wrong foods, save calories, and thus lose weight.

Note that all my smoothies and juices are fast fuels, with the exception of these slow-fuel beverages:

Almond Delight Smoothie
Fuelin' Veggie Juice 2

SUNRISE SMOOTHIE

If you want to start your day with an infusion of nutrients, this smoothie does the trick—fiber and phytochemicals from blueberries, vitamin C from orange juice, and potassium from the banana, plus a jolt of protein powder. This is really a complete meal in a glass.

1 SERVING

⅓ cup frozen blueberries

½ cup orange juice

½ cup low-fat plain yogurt

1 banana

1 tablespoon chia seeds

1 scoop vanilla plant-based protein powder

5 ice cubes

Combine all ingredients in a blender. Blend until smooth.

NUTRITION PER SERVING | FAT: 10 GRAMS | CARBOHYDRATE: 80 GRAMS | PROTEIN: 36 GRAMS | TOTAL CALORIES: 554

BLUEBERRY DREAM SMOOTHIE

V

Using frozen berries in your smoothie keeps things nice and frosty. You also avoid the problem of having fresh berries go bad quickly. You can buy packages of unsweetened frozen berries, or freeze your own.

1 SERVING

½ cup frozen blueberries

½ banana

1 scoop vanilla plant-based protein powder

1¼ cups water

2 teaspoons liquid coconut oil

1 tablespoon agave syrup

1 teaspoon chia seeds

Combine all ingredients in a blender. Blend until smooth.

HOO-YA

FREEZING BANANAS

When a recipe calls for half a banana, or your bananas are starting to turn brown, peel them, put them in a plastic freezer bag, and pop them in your freezer. I keep a stash of frozen bananas in my freezer at all times. That way, they're ready for my smoothies. Because all of the banana is frozen, there's no need to add ice cubes for texture. You can do the same with berries and peaches.

NUTRITION PER SERVING | FAT: 15 GRAMS | CARBOHYDRATE: 42 GRAMS | PROTEIN: 28 GRAMS | TOTAL CALORIES: 415

STRAWBERRY SMOOTHIE

For me, a must-have smoothie ingredient is the chia seed. Packed with omega-3 fatty acids—along with fiber, calcium, and antioxidants—these native Mexican seeds are favored by all health-conscious eaters.

1 SERVING

2 scoops vanilla plant-based protein powder

2 tablespoons flaxseed oil

1/2 cup low-fat plain Greek yogurt

1/2 cup frozen or fresh strawberries

1 tablespoon chia seeds

1 cup water

Combine all ingredients in a blender. Blend until smooth.

NUTRITION PER SERVING | FAT: 11 GRAMS | CARBOHYDRATE: 29 GRAMS | PROTEIN: 75 GRAMS | TOTAL CALORIES: 515

PINEAPPLE POWER SMOOTHIE

I love this smoothie for its tropical taste but also for its digestion-soothing power. The main ingredient here is pineapple. The fruit is the key to fighting that bloated feeling because it's rich in bromelain, an enzyme that aids digestion.

1 SERVING

1 cup pineapple juice

4 strawberries

1/2 cup frozen pineapple chunks

1/2 banana

1 teaspoon low-fat plain Greek yogurt

1 scoop vanilla plant-based protein powder

2 teaspoons liquid coconut oil

Combine all ingredients in a blender and blend until smooth. Serve immediately.

NUTRITION PER SERVING | FAT: 12 GRAMS | CARBOHYDRATE: 73 GRAMS | PROTEIN: 33 GRAMS | TOTAL CALORIES: 532

PUMPKIN PROTEIN SMOOTHIE

This smoothie includes almond milk, which has grown in popularity lately and is a delicious alternative to dairy. The smoothie is not only tasty but super-nutritious, too. It has protein for muscle building, fast fuel in the form of a banana for energy, probiotics for digestive health, and vitamin A for healthy skin and eyes, strong immune function, and protection against free radicals.

1 SERVING

1/4 cup 100 percent pure pumpkin puree (not pie filling)

1/2 banana

1/4 cup plain Greek yogurt

1 scoop vanilla plant-based protein powder

1 teaspoon chia seeds

1 cup unsweetened vanilla almond milk

1 tablespoon agave syrup

Combine all ingredients in a blender. Blend until smooth.

HOO-YA

CHA-CHA-CHA CHIA!

Chia seeds have now become even more famous for their nutritional attributes than they ever were for sprouting "hair" on clay pets. Resembling a black sesame seed and possessing a nutty flavor, chia seeds are an excellent source of minerals, antioxidants, fiber, and beneficial fats.

And they sure are versatile. You can eat them with cereal, mixed in yogurt, sprinkled over salads, and blended in smoothies. Usually you just eat them whole, but you can grind them and add to any flour-based or grain dish. You can purchase chia seeds at natural foods stores, supermarkets, or online. They can be stored in the fridge or pantry.

NUTRITION PER SERVING | FAT: 13 GRAMS | CARBOHYDRATE: 52 GRAMS | PROTEIN: 32 GRAMS | TOTAL CALORIES: 453

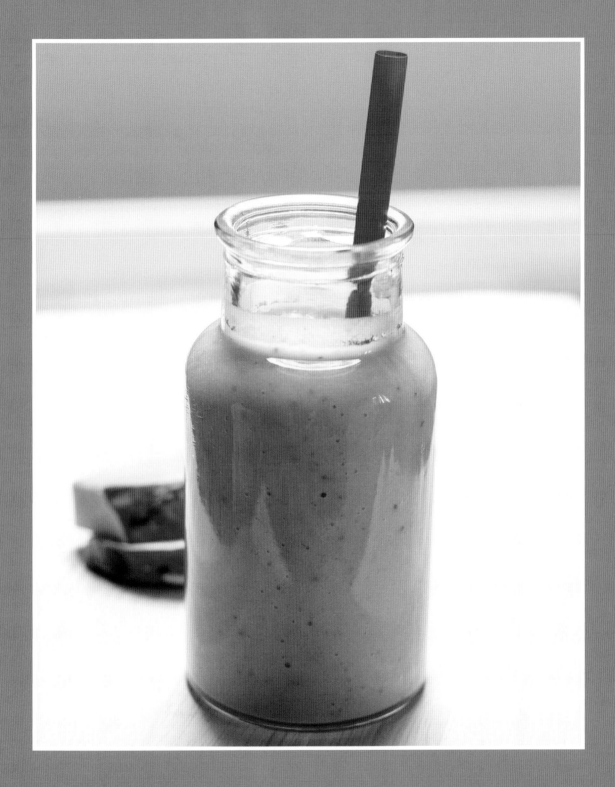

STRAWBERRY AND PINEAPPLE SMOOTHIE

V

I love the taste of the tropics, and this smoothie delivers it with the addition of banana and pineapple. It's loaded with protein, too, thanks to the triple whammy of almonds, almond milk, and protein powder.

1 SERVING

1 banana

1/2 cup frozen pineapple chunks

1 scoop vanilla plant-based protein powder

1/2 cup frozen strawberries

1 tablespoon chopped almonds

1/2 cup almond milk

1/2 cup water

Combine all ingredients in a blender. Blend until smooth.

NUTRITION PER SERVING | FAT: 18 GRAMS | CARBOHYDRATE: 66 GRAMS | PROTEIN: 34 GRAMS | TOTAL CALORIES: 562

PEACH PIE SMOOTHIE

If you love peach pie but don't love the calories it delivers, here's a luscious alternative. Trust me when I tell you it is truly a peach pie in a glass, and the Greek yogurt gives it an à la mode touch.

1 SERVING

1/2 cup fat-free plain Greek yogurt

3/4 cup frozen peaches

1 cup low-fat milk

1 tablespoon chopped almonds

2 scoops vanilla plant-based protein powder

1/2 teaspoon vanilla extract

1/2 teaspoon cinnamon

1/4 teaspoon ground nutmeg

1/2 tablespoon agave syrup

10 ice cubes

Combine all ingredients in a blender. Blend until smooth.

NUTRITION PER SERVING | FAT: 10 GRAMS | CARBOHYDRATE: 54 GRAMS | PROTEIN: 60 GRAMS | TOTAL CALORIES: 546

GREEN ZEN SMOOTHIE

V

We all know we should eat more greens, but sometimes it's hard to fit them into our diets. Smoothie to the rescue! Accented by fruit, green smoothies like this one are naturally sweet. They make me feel totally energized afterward.

1 SERVING

2 cups spinach, thawed from frozen

1 cup frozen strawberries

1 cup almond milk

1 cup frozen mango chunks

2 scoops vanilla plant-based protein powder

½ banana

1 teaspoon vanilla extract

2 teaspoons agave syrup

1 teaspoon chia seeds

1 teaspoon liquid coconut oil

Combine all ingredients in a blender. Blend until smooth.

HOO-YA

HOW TO EAT MORE GREENS

I love green leafy vegetables and try to eat them daily. Green leafy vegetables are full of health-protective phytochemicals, vitamins, minerals, and fiber. So beneficial are these veggies that I recommend incorporating at least 3 cups of cooked greens (or 6 cups raw) in your diet every week, or more.

That sounds like a lot of lettuce, kale, spinach, and other greens! But the good news is that there are ways to get your greens besides just salads and cooked-greens side dishes. For example:

- Toss a handful of spinach or kale in your smoothies.
- Drape piles of spinach over your pizzas.
- Make sure your sandwiches or wraps are filled to the brim with green lettuces or spinach leaves.
- Blend cooked spinach or kale into your mashed potatoes.
- Bake greens such as spinach or kale into meatloaf.
- Toss greens into soups.

These are just a few ideas. Let your culinary creativity go wild, and you'll easily get enough greens to bolster your health.

| NUTRITION PER SERVING | FAT: 16 GRAMS | CARBOHYDRATE: 64 GRAMS | PROTEIN: 32 GRAMS | TOTAL CALORIES: 528 |

THE HULK SMOOTHIE

This smoothie combines super-greens like spinach with sweet green fruits like apples and pears, plus a little ice cream for good measure! It's so delicious, you won't even know you're eating your veggies.

1 SERVING

2 scoops vanilla plant-based protein powder

1 stalk celery, chopped

¾ cup tightly packed spinach

½ green apple

1 kiwi, peeled and sliced

½ green pear, chopped

½ cucumber, peeled and chopped

1 tablespoon vanilla ice cream or Greek yogurt

2 tablespoons chopped almonds

5 ice cubes

Combine all ingredients in a blender. Blend until smooth. If it's too thick, add a little water.

NUTRITION PER SERVING | FAT: 22 GRAMS | CARBOHYDRATE: 80 GRAMS | PROTEIN: 58 GRAMS | TOTAL CALORIES: 710

APPLE MELONTINI SMOOTHIE

Thick with delicious fruit and vitamin A–pumped carrots, this smoothie is a perfect fast fuel for breakfast or refueling after a good workout. It's protein-rich, too, thanks to the addition of yogurt and protein powder.

1 SERVING

2 apples, cored and chopped

1 cup chopped cantaloupe

5 tablespoons plain Greek yogurt

1/2 carrot, chopped

1/2 cup strawberries

1 scoop plain plant-based protein powder

Combine all ingredients in a blender. Blend until smooth. Serve immediately.

NUTRITION PER SERVING | FAT: 3 GRAMS | CARBOHYDRATE: 83 GRAMS | PROTEIN: 28 GRAMS | TOTAL CALORIES: 471

MANGO GINGER SMOOTHIE

Here's a recipe inspired by a cool, refreshing drink that I sipped on a tropical beach. High in fiber, this smoothie is packed with antioxidants and protein to help you stay energized all day.

1 SERVING

1 cup frozen mango chunks

1/3 cup frozen pineapple chunks

1/2 cup chopped carrots

1 teaspoon grated ginger

4 tablespoons plain low-fat Greek yogurt

1 scoop plain plant-based protein powder

Combine all ingredients in a blender. Blend until smooth.

NUTRITION PER SERVING | FAT: 3 GRAMS | CARBOHYDRATE: 46 GRAMS | PROTEIN: 25 GRAMS | TOTAL CALORIES: 311

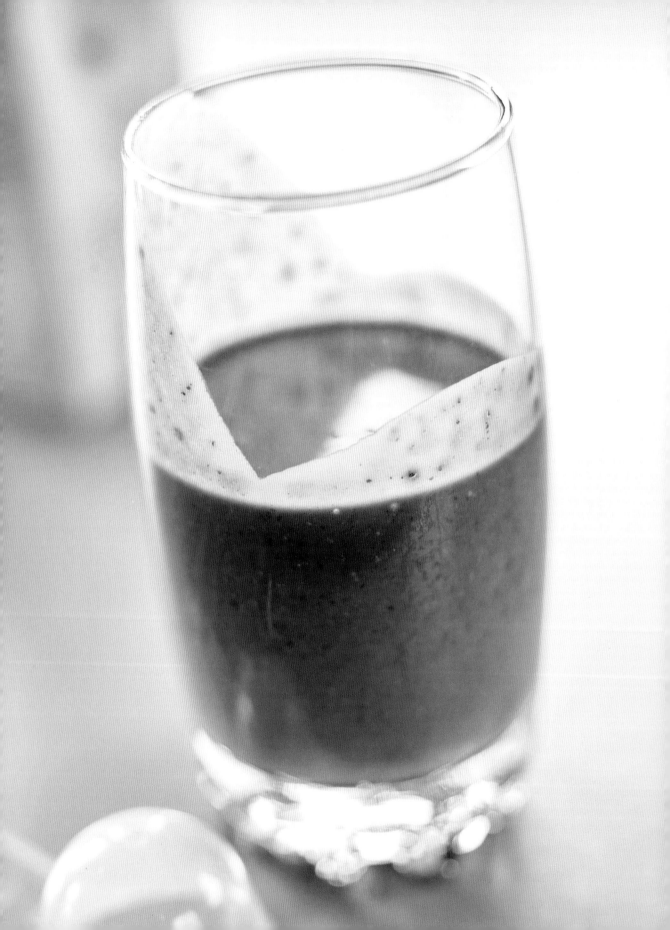

ALMOND DELIGHT SMOOTHIE

V

Whiz together chocolate protein powder, almond milk, and coconut oil, and you've practically got dessert! But even though this sounds a bit like the candy bar that inspired it, it's a totally healthful indulgence.

1 SERVING

1 cup unsweetened almond milk

1 tablespoon almond butter

2 scoops chocolate plant-based protein powder

1 teaspoon chia seeds

1 teaspoon liquid coconut oil

Combine all ingredients in a blender and blend until smooth. Serve immediately.

NUTRITION PER SERVING | FAT: 20 GRAMS | CARBOHYDRATE: 10 GRAMS | PROTEIN: 31 GRAMS | TOTAL CALORIES: 344

GREEN WITH ENVY JUICE

V

If you don't like to swallow vitamin pills, juicing is a great alternative. Depending on the fruits and veggies you juice, you're creating a drinkable vitamin supplement in a glass. This recipe has vitamin-packed greens, fiber, digestion-friendly ginger, and a blast of protein and good fat—a thoroughly healthful energy drink.

1 SERVING

1 cucumber

2 green apples

2 stalks celery

1 cup tightly packed spinach

1-inch piece ginger

2 leaves kale

1 scoop plain plant-based protein powder

1/2 tablespoon liquid coconut oil

Add all ingredients to juicer except the coconut oil. Juice according to the manufacturer's direction. Once juiced, add coconut oil and mix well.

NUTRITION PER SERVING | FAT: 9 GRAMS | CARBOHYDRATE: 75 GRAMS | PROTEIN: 19 GRAMS | TOTAL CALORIES: 457

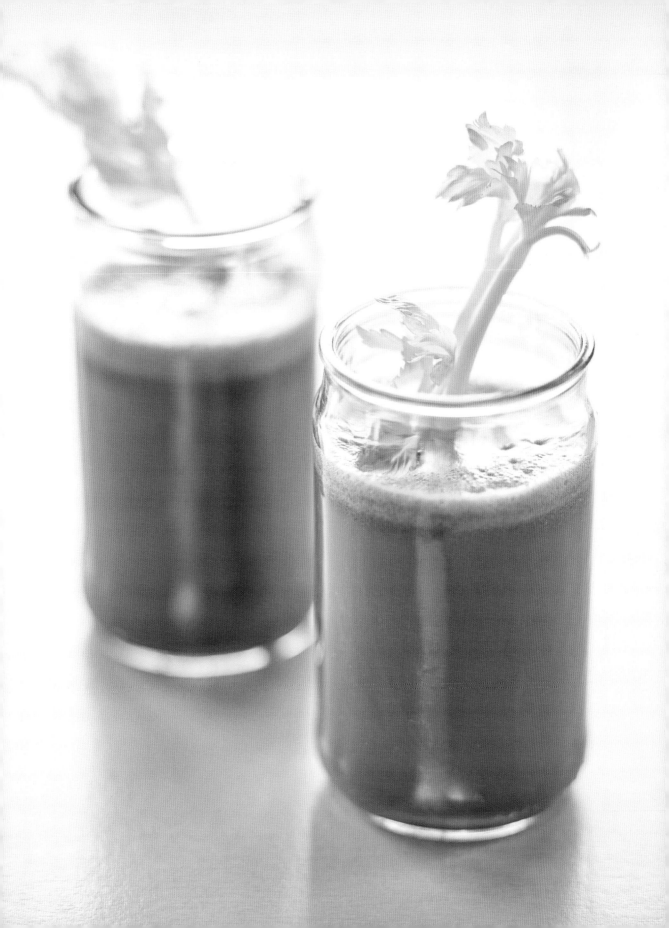

BLENDED SUPER JUICE

V

I call this Super Juice because it contains superior fuels that your body will love: apple for fiber, almonds and protein powder for protein, avocado for healthful fat, pineapple for the digestion-friendly bromelain, and vitamin-loaded greens. All of this is blended, too—no juicer required. Plus, this juice makes a delicious fast-fuel meal or snack. It just doesn't get much better than this!

2 SERVINGS

1 apple, cored and chopped

1 cup tightly packed spinach

1/2 avocado

1/4 cup almonds

11/2 cups water

2 tablespoons lemon juice

1/2 cup pineapple juice

1/2 cucumber

11/2 cups tightly packed collard greens

1 scoop plain plant-based protein powder

Combine all ingredients in a blender. Blend until smooth.

NUTRITION PER SERVING | FAT: 13 GRAMS | CARBOHYDRATE: 40 GRAMS | PROTEIN: 20 GRAMS | TOTAL CALORIES: 357

GREEN GODDESS SMOOTHIE

V

Here's a super-delicious, super-healthful juice, and you don't even need a juicer to make it. Sweetened by the tropical combination of banana and coconut water, this juice whizzes together three of the most nutritious greens on the planet.

1 SERVING

1 cup kale

1 cup tightly packed baby spinach

1/2 cucumber, chopped

1/2 cup coconut water

1 broccoli head, chopped

1/2 banana

1/2 tablespoon liquid coconut oil

1 scoop vanilla plant-based protein powder.

Combine all ingredients in a blender. Blend until smooth.

NUTRITION PER SERVING   FAT: 8 GRAMS   CARBOHYDRATE: 64 GRAMS   PROTEIN: 19 GRAMS   TOTAL CALORIES: 348

FUELIN' VEGGIE JUICE 2

V

Here's my version of bottled V-8 and similar products. Although you blend it, it is still technically a juice, but one that preserves all the fiber in the vegetables. Blended juices like this one are so easy to make, and cleanup is a breeze.

2 SERVINGS

2 cups tomato juice

1 cucumber, chopped

1/2 bell pepper, chopped

1/2 cup tightly packed spinach

2 dill stems, chopped

1 tablespoon lemon juice

1 scoop unflavored plant-based protein powder

1/2 tablespoon avocado oil

1/2 cup chopped carrots

Pinch salt

Mint leaves, for garnish

Combine all ingredients except the mint in a blender. Blend until smooth. Garnish with mint leaves.

NUTRITION PER SERVING | FAT: 8 GRAMS | CARBOHYDRATE: 25 GRAMS | PROTEIN: 15 GRAMS | TOTAL CALORIES: 232

JUST BEET IT JUICE

V

Want to boost your exercise or athletic endurance? Try beet juice. It has a high level of natural nitrate, which has been shown clinically to boost performance. Scientists aren't exactly sure how beet juice works like this, but they suspect that the more nitric oxide in your body, a by-product of nitrate, the more you can exercise with less oxygen. Spinach (also found in this recipe) is high in dietary nitrate, too. In terms of taste, this juice is naturally sweet with a slight earthy taste.

1 SERVING

1/2 cup peeled, diced beets

1/2 tablespoon grated ginger

3 large oranges

1 apple

1/2 cup chopped carrots

1 handful spinach

1 stalk celery

1 scoop plain plant-based protein powder

1/2 tablespoon liquid coconut oil

One by one, run the fruits and vegetables through the juicer. Whisk in the protein powder and oil until the powder dissolves.

NUTRITION PER SERVING | FAT: 9 GRAMS | CARBOHYDRATE: 68 GRAMS | PROTEIN: 35 GRAMS | TOTAL CALORIES: 493

RED GRAPEFRUIT JUICE

V

Grapefruit contains an antioxidant called naringin that apparently blocks the uptake of fatty acids into cells and reduces the body's ability to store carbohydrates. These attributes make grapefruit a potential fat burner. This recipe combines grapefruit with other fruits and veggies, all of which are high in fiber (another known fat burner).

1 SERVING

2 grapefruits, peeled and white pith removed

2-inch beet, peeled

2 stalks celery

1/2 apple

1 scoop plain plant-based protein powder

One by one, run the first four ingredients through the juicer. Whisk in the protein powder.

NUTRITION PER SERVING | FAT: 2 GRAMS | CARBOHYDRATE: 65 GRAMS | PROTEIN: 20 GRAMS | TOTAL CALORIES: 358

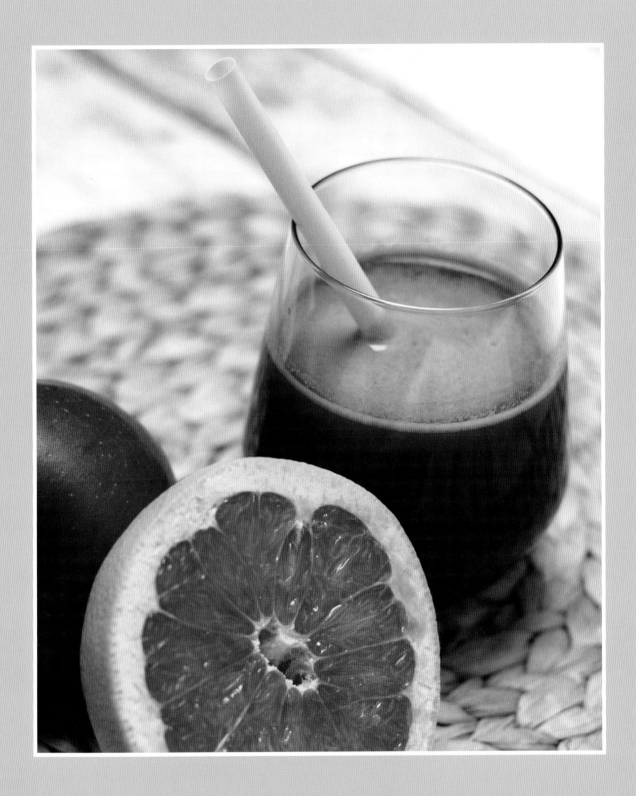

RASPBERRY TANG JUICE

V

This delicious fast-fuel juice has a very fruity yet tangy taste. The main act is raspberries—a health star that is low in calories, high in fiber, and loaded with phyto-nutrients.

1 SERVING

11/2 cups raspberries

1 large apple, cored and chopped

1/2 cucumber, chopped

1 orange, peeled and seeded

1/2 tablespoon liquid coconut oil

1 scoop plain plant-based protein powder

Combine all ingredients in a blender. Blend until smooth.

NUTRITION PER SERVING | FAT: 8 GRAMS | CARBOHYDRATE: 80 GRAMS | PROTEIN: 26 GRAMS | TOTAL CALORIES: 497

WATERMELON BASIL JUICE

V

I've always loved watermelon. Unlike fattening desserts, which you should limit, you can gorge on watermelon for dessert until it runs out. Here, I've taken advantage of its natural sweetness to make a refreshing juice. There's clearly a lot you can do with watermelon besides just chomping on slices and spitting out the seeds!

1 SERVING

1 apple, cored and chopped
1 cup seedless watermelon chunks
1/3 cup strawberries
1/2 cup chopped carrots

1/2 tablespoon liquid coconut oil
1 scoop plain plant-based protein powder
Handful of chopped fresh basil

Add fruits and carrots into juicer or blender and blend until smooth. Whisk in the oil, protein powder, and basil until the powder dissolves.

NUTRITION PER SERVING | FAT: 8 GRAMS | CARBOHYDRATE: 55 GRAMS | PROTEIN: 25 GRAMS | TOTAL CALORIES: 392

Chapter 6

Fast-Fuel Desserts

On my eating plan, you can eat desserts. I'm sure that's good news for anyone with a sweet tooth. When creating these desserts, I relied on fruits, natural sweeteners, and whole grains, making all of these recipes fast fuels.

Each recipe makes more than one serving. I recommend that you prepare these big batches and refrigerate or freeze them so that you always have a treat on hand. Enjoy!

NO-BAKE CHOCOLATE APPLE OATMEAL COOKIES

V

This is one of the easiest cookie recipes you can make—a quick one-pan wonder that requires no baking. It's so good that you'll be tempted to eat the batter right out of the pan, but try to resist, because once they cool and set, they are even better! These delicious treats count as fast fuels.

12 SERVINGS

2 tablespoons agave syrup

2 tablespoons coconut oil

½ cup light coconut milk

2 scoops chocolate plant-based protein powder

3 cups rolled oats

¼ teaspoon salt

1 teaspoon vanilla extract

½ cup chopped dried apples

Combine agave, coconut oil, coconut milk, and protein powder in a large pan and boil 3–5 minutes. Stir in oats, salt, vanilla extract, and apple.

Drop spoonfuls of batter onto a parchment-paper-lined baking sheet. Let cool for 10–15 minutes, until cookies set; alternatively, refrigerate until set.

NUTRITION PER SERVING FAT: 5 GRAMS | CARBOHYDRATE: 19 GRAMS | PROTEIN: 9 GRAMS | TOTAL CALORIES: 157

NO-BAKE ALMOND BUTTER SQUARES

Give your oven a break with these no-bake fast-fuel treats. They're great for time-strapped cooks, too—they'll get you in and out of the kitchen in minimum time.

24 SERVINGS

½ cup agave syrup
1 cup almond butter

3 cups rolled oats

Combine agave and almond butter in a saucepan. Heat the mixture over medium heat until combined. Add the oats and mix well.

Coat a 9-by-9-inch baking pan with cooking spray. Pour mixture into pan and press it to the edges. Place in refrigerator until set. Keep squares stored in refrigerator to prevent melting.

NUTRITION PER SERVING FAT: 6 GRAMS CARBOHYDRATE: 13 GRAMS PROTEIN: 4 GRAMS TOTAL CALORIES: 122

BANANA BLUEBERRY COOKIES

V

One of the best-kept baking secrets for making no-sugar desserts is to use pitted dates as the fill-in for sugar. Dates are naturally sweet and full of nutrients. Plus, they act like a binder, holding all the other ingredients together. The rolled oats and fruit make these cookies a delectable fast-fuel dessert.

24 SERVINGS

3 bananas

2 cups rolled oats

1/2 cup dried blueberries

5 dates, pitted and chopped

2 tablespoons coconut oil

1 teaspoon vanilla extract

2 tablespoons flaxseeds

1 teaspoon nutmeg

1 teaspoon cinnamon

Preheat oven to 350 degrees. Coat a baking sheet with cooking spray.

In a large bowl, mash the bananas. Stir in the remaining ingredients. Mix well and let mixture set for 15 minutes.

Spoon by teaspoonfuls onto the baking sheet. Bake for 20 minutes, until lightly brown.

NUTRITION PER SERVING | FAT: 3 GRAMS | CARBOHYDRATE: 15 GRAMS | PROTEIN: 1 GRAM | TOTAL CALORIES: 82

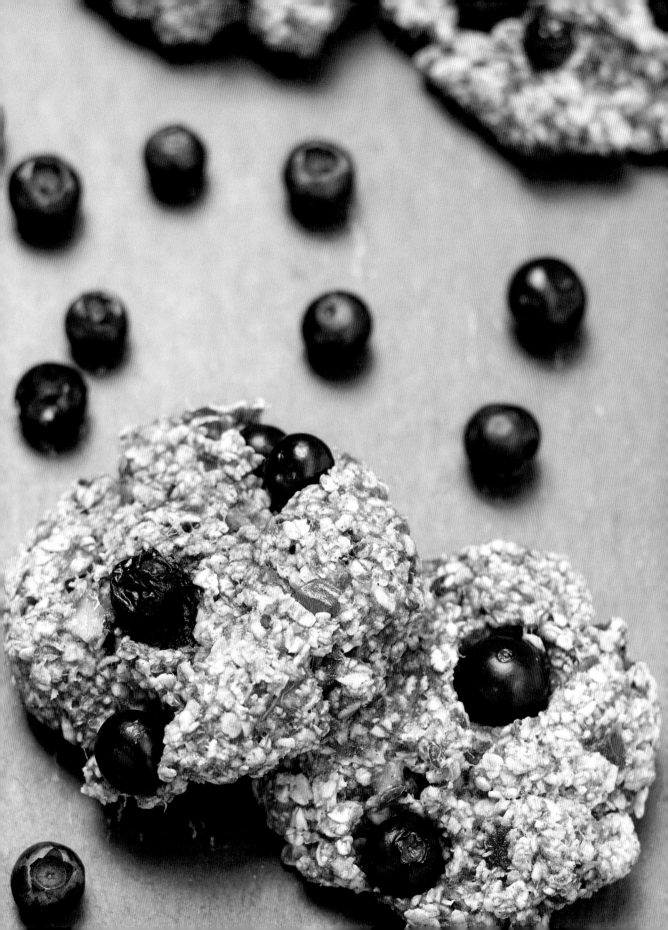

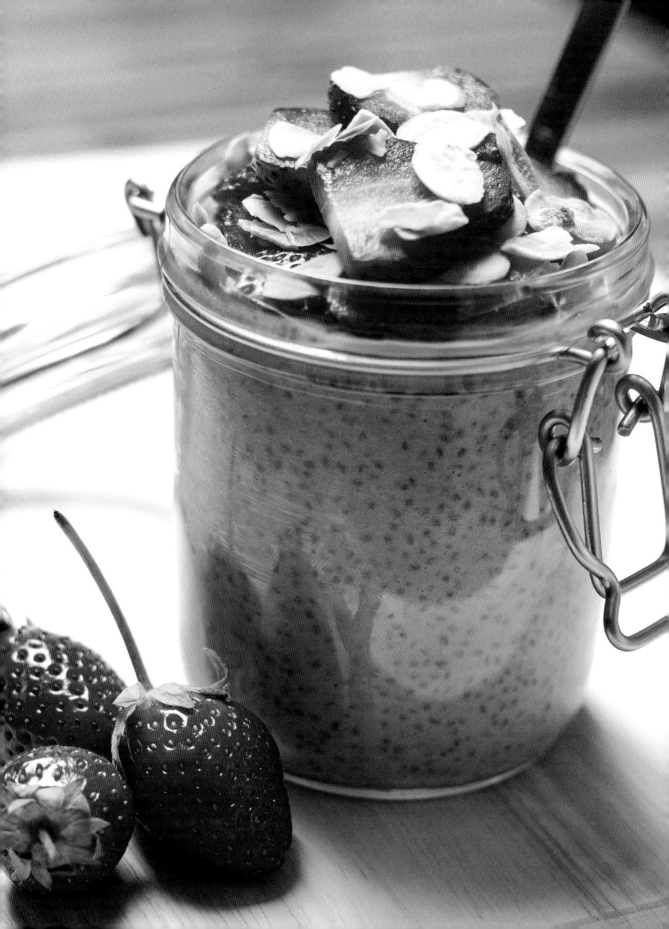

CHOCOLATE STRAWBERRY CHIA PUDDING

V

A key ingredient in this delicious pudding is the chia seed, a member of the mint family that is native to Mexico and Guatemala. Dating back to the Aztecs, chia seeds were an important food crop in ancient times, but they didn't become known in North America until about thirty years ago. They make a terrific thickener for healthful puddings like this fast fuel because they swell up when mixed with liquid.

4 SERVINGS

⅓ cup chia seeds

2 scoops chocolate plant-based protein powder

2–4 tablespoons agave syrup

1½ cups coconut milk

½ teaspoon cinnamon

¼ teaspoon salt

½ teaspoon vanilla extract

2 tablespoons sliced almonds

1 cup sliced strawberries

In a bowl, combine the chia seeds, protein powder, agave syrup, coconut milk, cinnamon, salt, and vanilla extract. Divide the pudding between four small mason jars or other containers. Cover the containers and place in the refrigerator for a few hours until the pudding thickens, or overnight.

Serve chilled with almonds and strawberries.

NUTRITION PER SERVING | FAT: 12 GRAMS | CARBOHYDRATE: 31 GRAMS | PROTEIN: 12 GRAMS | TOTAL CALORIES: 280

PROTEIN CARROT CAKE BITES

V

This fast-fuel dessert is a remake of classic carrot cake, except that it's not baked. Plus, it's wheat- and dairy-free. Its flavor and texture are accented by the assertive presence of coconut, and protein powder makes it a great recipe for post-workout refueling.

40 BALLS

1 cup unsweetened shredded coconut

6 dates, pitted

¾ cup walnuts

½ cup shredded carrots

2 tablespoons agave syrup

2 teaspoons vanilla extract

¼ cup plain plant-based protein powder

½ teaspoon nutmeg

1 teaspoon cinnamon

¼ teaspoon cloves

Combine ½ cup shredded coconut with the other 9 ingredients in a food processor. Process until all ingredients are combined well.

Place the remaining coconut in a shallow bowl. Take a small amount of the date mixture and form a bite-size ball. Roll the ball in the reserved coconut. Place the balls on a baking sheet, cover, and refrigerate for a few hours or overnight. The balls are ready to eat once they are firm.

| NUTRITION PER SERVING | FAT: 2 GRAMS | CARBOHYDRATE: 4 GRAMS | PROTEIN: 2 GRAM | TOTAL CALORIES: 42 |

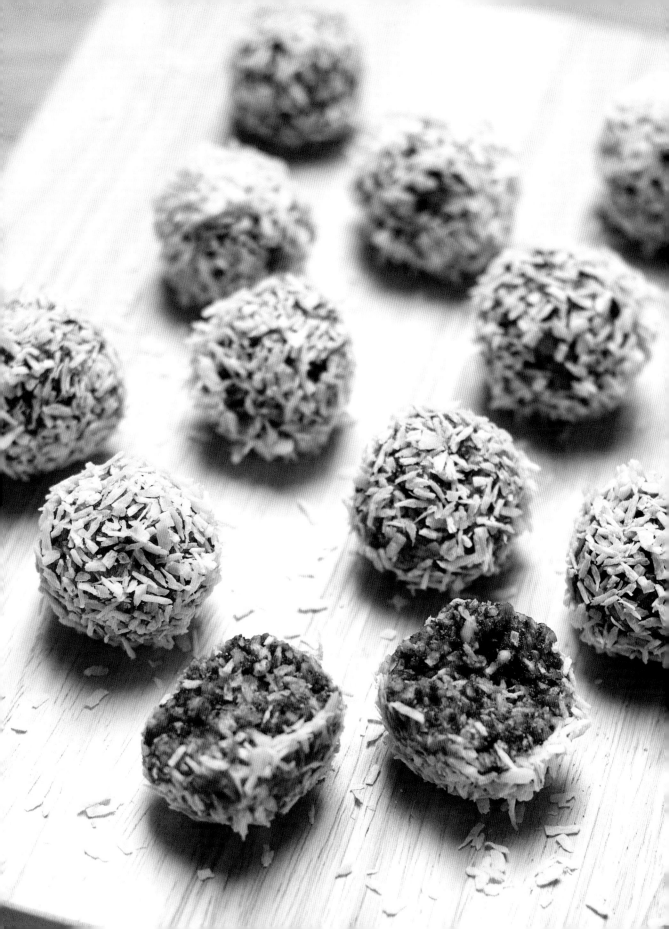

NO-BAKE ALMOND BUTTER BANANA BITES

V

What makes this recipe special is the combination of melted chocolate and sliced bananas, teamed up with chopped almonds. Everyone will go bananas over the taste of these fast-fuel bites.

18 SERVINGS

3 bananas, sliced
1/2 cup almond butter

11/2 cups dark chocolate chips
1/4 cup chopped almonds

Place half the sliced bananas on a baking sheet. Spoon a dab of almond butter on top of each banana slice, and top with another banana slice to make a sandwich. Place in the freezer for 3 hours or until firm.

In a saucepan over medium-low heat, heat chocolate chips and stir until smooth. Hold banana sandwiches between two forks and dip them in the melted chocolate, one by one, until completely covered. Sprinkle the almonds on top, place the bananas back on the baking tray, and let the chocolate set. Keep bananas bites in the refrigerator or freezer.

NUTRITION PER SERVING | FAT: 7 GRAMS | CARBOHYDRATE: 13 GRAMS | PROTEIN: 5 GRAMS | TOTAL CALORIES: 135

CHOCOLATE BANANA PROTEIN CUPCAKES

Ah . . . cupcakes. What comfort food could be better? I've creatively added lots of protein to this dish, with eggs, egg whites, protein powder, and walnuts. Enjoy these fast-fuel delights anytime—for breakfast, as a snack, or for dessert.

12 SERVINGS

1 cup walnuts

3 large eggs

2 egg whites

11/4 cups mashed banana

1 cup chocolate plant-based protein powder

1/4 teaspoon salt

1/2 teaspoon vanilla extract

1 teaspoon baking powder

Preheat oven to 325 degrees. Coat a 12-cup muffin tin with cooking spray.

In a food processor, pulse the walnuts until finely chopped. Add the eggs, egg whites, banana, protein powder, salt, vanilla extract, and baking powder. Blend until smooth.

Pour mixture into muffin cups and bake 20–25 minutes, until center is set. Completely cool cupcakes before removing from pan. You can tightly wrap the cupcakes individually in plastic wrap and store them in the refrigerator or in an airtight container in the freezer.

NUTRITION PER SERVING | FAT: 8 GRAMS | CARBOHYDRATE: 10 GRAMS | PROTEIN: 19 GRAMS | TOTAL CALORIES: 158

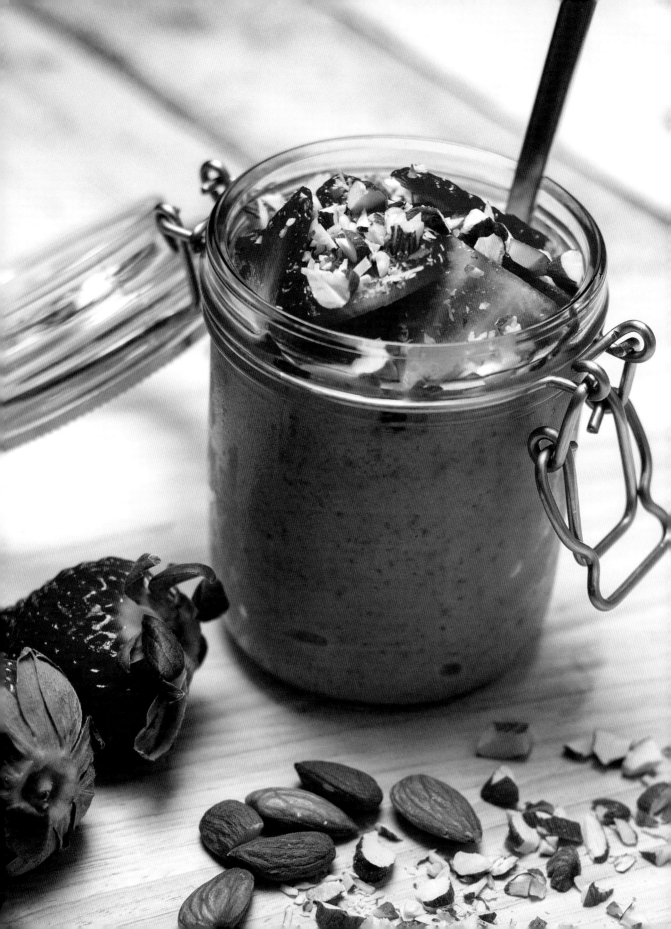

STRAWBERRY FROZEN YOGURT

Frozen yogurt is generally more healthful than ice cream, because it is lower in fat and has more protein and calcium, but some commercial varieties are high in sugar and may have other additives you could do without. The best alternative is to make it yourself, and this super-easy fast-fuel recipe shows you how.

1 SERVING

1 cup frozen strawberries
1/4 cup low-fat plain Greek yogurt
1/2 scoop vanilla plant-based protein powder

1/2 tablespoon lemon juice
1 tablespoon agave syrup
1/2 tablespoon chopped almonds

Combine all ingredients except the almonds in a blender and blend until smooth and creamy. Stir in the almonds and serve immediately, or transfer to an airtight container and freeze.

NUTRITION PER SERVING | FAT: 5 GRAMS | CARBOHYDRATE: 24 GRAMS | PROTEIN: 10 GRAMS | TOTAL CALORIES: 181

SUNSHINE SORBET

V

Sorbet is a smooth water ice, said to be the first iced dessert in history. Sorbets are the perfect refreshing summer dessert. Plus, they're simple and relatively quick to assemble with a wide variety of fruits. Traditionally, sorbets are made with ice cream machines, but using a blender and frozen fruit produces results that are just as fine without the fuss. Enjoy this fruit fast fuel.

1 SERVING

1/2 cup chopped mango
1 banana, frozen

1 tablespoon chopped walnuts

Combine the mango and banana in a blender. Blend until smooth. Garnish with walnuts. Serve immediately, or transfer to an airtight container and freeze.

NUTRITION PER SERVING | FAT: 10 GRAMS | CARBOHYDRATE: 44 GRAMS | PROTEIN: 4 GRAMS | TOTAL CALORIES: 282

Chapter 7

Block Out Your Meals

Lots of *You Are Your Own Gym* and *Body Fuel* fans tell me that they like things really spelled out—leaving too many details up in the air can lead to overeating or even undernourishment. If this describes you, this section will solve your issues. Here I'm giving you six weeks of menus using recipes in this book as well as some simple preparations of ingredients you'll have on hand if you are also following the weekly shopping lists I've provided for each weekly menu.

Planning meals is a cinch—all you do is select a fast-fuel recipe or a slow-fuel recipe and slot it into the meal design each day. This is an easy-to-follow plan, and you can do it to the letter, down to the very last snack.

Or you can be your own nutritionist, decide on your own food choices by selecting foods from fast-fuel and slow-fuel lists and designing your meals to your preferences. Here's an example.

BLOCK 3 DAY

BREAKFAST (FAST FUEL)

2 slices Canadian bacon

11/4 cups packaged cereal such as Special K or a high-fiber cereal such as
   raisin bran or Fiber One

1 cup almond milk

LUNCH (FAST FUEL)

Grilled chicken breast (6–8 ounces for men, 3–5 ounces for women)

Brown rice, cooked (1 cup for men, 1/2 cup for women)

Tossed salad with 1–2 tablespoons low-fat salad dressing

DINNER (FAST FUEL)

Roast beef, such as eye round (6–8 ounces for men, 3–5 ounces for women)

Asparagus sautéed in 1 tablespoon olive oil

1 baked potato, topped with 1–2 tablespoons nonfat sour cream if desired

SNACK 1 (FAST FUEL)

Banana

SNACK 2 (SLOW FUEL)

1/2 chicken breast

Raw cut-up slow-fuel veggies

BLOCK 2 DAY

BREAKFAST (FAST FUEL)

Soft-boiled eggs (4 for men, 2 for women)
Oatmeal with berries

LUNCH (FAST FUEL)

Cooked lean ground beef, cooked kidney beans (1 cup for men, 1/2 cup for women), tomato
 sauce, and spices, mixed together to make a quick chili

DINNER (SLOW FUEL)

Grilled or baked salmon (6–8 ounces for men, 3–5 ounces for women)
Kale sautéed in 1 tablespoon olive oil
Wax beans

SNACK 1 (SLOW FUEL)

1 hard-boiled egg
Handful of almonds

SNACK 2 (SLOW FUEL)

1/2 grilled chicken breast
Cut-up raw cauliflower

BLOCK 1 DAY

BREAKFAST (FAST FUEL)

Turkey sausage links or patties (4 pieces for men, 2 pieces for women), pan-fried
Whole-grain or sprouted-grain toast (2 slices for men, 1 slice for women), with all-fruit jam if
  desired

LUNCH (SLOW FUEL)

Salad bar: 1–2 cups fresh greens, 1/2 cup kidney beans or chickpeas, tomato slices, chopped
  green bell peppers, 1 tablespoon sunflower seeds, 1–2 tablespoons low-fat salad dressing

DINNER (SLOW FUEL)

Asian takeout of mixed steamed vegetables and shrimp (2 cups for men, 1 cup for women)

SNACK 1 (SLOW FUEL)

1 hard-boiled egg
Handful of almonds

SNACK 2 (SLOW FUEL)

1/2 piece grilled chicken breast
1 cup kale chips

If you're a vegan or vegetarian, see page 236—here you'll find 3 weeks of calorie-cycling menus tailored to your diet.

A note about serving sizes: You can adjust the serving sizes up or down, depending on your goal. For example, if you're trying to build mass or maintain your weight, make your servings larger than what is stated in the recipe, so that you consume more growth-producing calories. On the other hand, if you're intent on losing weight and obtaining lean muscle definition, eat smaller portions than what is listed in each recipe.

MEAL DESIGN FOR BLOCK 3

Breakfast Pattern: protein + 1 serving fast-fuel carb

Lunch Pattern: protein + 1 serving fast-fuel carb and liberal amounts of slow-fuel carbs

Dinner Pattern: protein + 1 serving fast-fuel carb and liberal amounts of slow-fuel carbs

Snack Pattern (1 midmorning, 1 midafternoon): protein + nuts or seeds or a slow-fuel carb; as your second snack, have a protein + a fast-fuel carb. This pattern should be eaten following a workout.

Stay on Block 3 for 3 weeks.

BLOCK 3 WEEK 1 SAMPLE MENU (4 FAST FUELS DAILY)

DAY 1

BREAKFAST (FAST FUEL)

Baked Egg in a Hole (page 25)

LUNCH (FAST FUEL)

Salmon Salad Sandwich (page 35)

DINNER (FAST FUEL)

Ginger Beef (page 83)

SNACK 1 (FAST FUEL)

The Hulk Smoothie (page 165)

SNACK 2 (SLOW FUEL)

Hard-boiled eggs (3–4 for men, 1–2 for women)
Handful of almonds

DAY 2

BREAKFAST (FAST FUEL)

Soft-boiled eggs (3–4 for men, 1–2 for women)
Oatmeal with berries (1 cup for men, 1/2 cup for women)

LUNCH (FAST FUEL)

Chicken Orzo Salad (page 38)

DINNER (FAST FUEL)

Coriander Baked Salmon (page 60)

SNACK 1 (SLOW FUEL)

1/2 grilled chicken breast
8 ounces **Fuelin' Veggie Juice 2 (page 174)**

SNACK 2 (FAST FUEL)

Peach Pie Smoothie (page 163)

DAY 3

BREAKFAST (FAST FUEL)

Sunrise Egg Muffin (page 30)

LUNCH (FAST FUEL)

Guilt-Free Sloppy Joe (page 49)

DINNER (FAST FUEL)

Slow Cooker Indian Lamb Curry (page 85)

SNACK 1 (SLOW FUEL)

1/2 chicken breast
Raw cut-up slow-fuel veggies

SNACK 2 (FAST FUEL)

Green Goddess Smoothie (page 173)

DAY 4

BREAKFAST (FAST FUEL)

Complete Morning Glory (page 26)

LUNCH (FAST FUEL)

Lean ground beef patty (6–8 ounces for men,
 3–5 ounces for women)
Tossed salad with 1–2 tablespoons low-fat
 salad dressing
Black beans, cooked (1 cup for men, 1/2 cup
 for women)

DINNER (FAST FUEL)

Spicy Shrimp and Wild Rice (page 61)

SNACK 1 (SLOW FUEL)

Hard-boiled eggs (3–4 for men, 1–2 for
 women)
Handful of almonds

SNACK 2 (FAST FUEL)

**Chocolate Banana Protein Cupcakes
 (page 191)**

DAY 5

BREAKFAST (FAST FUEL)

Hangover Breakfast Sandwich (page 32)

LUNCH (FAST FUEL)

Mediterranean Chicken Wraps (page 47)

DINNER (FAST FUEL)

2 broiled veal chops (6–8 ounces for men, 3–5 ounces for women), topped with no-sugar-added pasta sauce

Zucchini sautéed in 1 tablespoon olive oil

Whole-wheat pasta, cooked (1 cup for men, 1/2 cup for women)

SNACK 1 (SLOW FUEL)

Handful of almonds or walnuts

Raw cut-up slow-fuel veggies

SNACK 2 (FAST FUEL)

Blueberry Dream Smoothie (page 157)

DAY 6

BREAKFAST (FAST FUEL)

Broccoli and Goat Cheese Omelet with Toast (page 31)

LUNCH (FAST FUEL)

Tex-Mex Corn and Avocado Salad (page 50)

DINNER (FAST FUEL)

Five-Spice Pork Chops (page 87)

SNACK 1 (SLOW FUEL)

Stuffed Eggs (page 150)

SNACK 2 (FAST FUEL)

Strawberry Smoothie (page 158)

DAY 7

BREAKFAST (FAST FUEL)

Scrambled eggs (3–4 for men, 2 for women)
1 Roma tomato, sliced
Grits, cooked (1 cup for men, 1/2 cup for
   women)

LUNCH (FAST FUEL)

Chicken Kale Soup (page 45)

DINNER (FAST FUEL)

Ginger Sea Bass (page 59)

SNACK 1 (SLOW FUEL)

2–3 ounces tuna
1 cup kale chips

SNACK 2 (FAST FUEL)

Green Zen Smoothie (page 164)

VEGETABLES

1 bunch celery

1 red onion

2 white onions

1 large yellow onion

1 small head butter lettuce

Fresh ginger

1 garlic bulb

One 12-ounce package frozen Asian vegetables

1 bunch scallions

1 bag spinach

1 bag kale

1 bag mixed greens (for salads)

1 bag baby carrots

2–3 cucumbers

1 English cucumber

1 package carrots

1 bottle tomato juice

1 red bell pepper

1 green bell pepper

1 package fresh dill

1 package baby arugula

2 cups French green beans

1 package fresh mint

1 package fresh oregano

1 bunch cilantro

3 tomatoes

1 Roma tomato

1 package grape tomatoes

1 package cherry tomatoes

One 14.5-ounce can diced tomatoes

1 bunch broccoli

3–4 zucchini

Two 15-ounce cans black beans

One 15-ounce can corn

2 cups fingerling potatoes

1 package fresh rosemary

1 bunch asparagus

1 red or green chile

1 bag frozen spinach

FRUITS

1 green apple

1 green pear

1 kiwi

1 lemon

2 tangerines

1 bag frozen peaches

1 bag frozen strawberries

1 bag frozen blueberries

1 bag frozen mango

1 small carton fresh strawberries

1 small carton fresh blueberries

2 avocados

4–5 bananas

POULTRY

1 rotisserie chicken

11/2 pounds ground turkey

1 package turkey links, sausage flavored

1 package turkey bacon

SEAFOOD

Two 4-ounce cans salmon packed in water

Six 3-ounce salmon fillets

Three 5-ounce cans tuna packed in water

Four 6-ounce wild sea bass fillets

MEATS

1 package bacon

1 package Canadian bacon

16 ounces tri-tip or sirloin steak

2 pounds lamb

1 package lean ground beef

2 veal chops

EGGS AND DAIRY

4 dozen eggs

1 carton grated Parmesan cheese

1 pint vanilla ice cream

1 package goat cheese

1 package feta cheese

One 16-ounce carton low-fat plain Greek yogurt

1 small carton low-fat milk

1 carton unsweetened almond milk

BREADS, CEREALS, PASTA, AND GRAINS

Several packages brown rice

1 package wild rice

Several packages whole-wheat orzo

1 loaf whole-wheat bread

1 large carton oatmeal

1 large carton grits

1 package whole-wheat English muffins

6 hamburger buns

1 package whole-wheat pasta

4 pork loin chops

NUTS AND SEEDS

Several packages raw almonds

1 large package chia seeds

1 package walnuts

1 package hemp seeds

MISCELLANEOUS

1 large jar low-fat mayonnaise

1 jar pesto sauce

1 jar Montreal steak seasoning

1 bottle low-sodium soy sauce

1 bottle lemon juice

1 bottle lime juice

1 jar coriander seeds

1 bottle avocado oil

1 large can tomato sauce

1 small can tomato paste

1 small bag all-purpose flour

1 jar mustard seeds

1 carton coconut water

1 jar pitted Kalamata olives

1 jar dill pickles

1 package kale chips

1 carton plain hummus

1 small package whole wheat crackers

BLOCK 3 WEEK 2 SAMPLE MENU (4 FAST FUELS DAILY)

DAY 8

BREAKFAST (FAST FUEL)

2 slices Canadian bacon
11/4 cups packaged cereal such as Special K
  or a high-fiber cereal like raisin bran or Fiber
  One
1 cup almond milk

LUNCH (FAST FUEL)

Chicken Curry Wraps (page 41)

DINNER (FAST FUEL)

Ginger Sea Bass (page 59)

SNACK 1 (FAST FUEL)

**Almond Butter and Jelly Rice Cakes
(page 96)**

SNACK 2 (SLOW FUEL)

Hard-boiled eggs (3–4 for men, 1–2 for
  women)
Handful of almonds

DAY 9

BREAKFAST (FAST FUEL)

Baked Egg in a Hole (page 25)

LUNCH (FAST FUEL)

**Chicken with Strawberries and Spinach
  Salad (page 51)**

DINNER (FAST FUEL)

Five-Spice Pork Chops (page 87)

SNACK 1 (SLOW FUEL)

1/2 grilled chicken breast
8 ounces **Fuelin' Veggie Juice 2 (page 174)**

SNACK 2 (FAST FUEL)

Pumpkin Protein Smoothie (page 160)

DAY 10

BREAKFAST (FAST FUEL)

Sunrise Smoothie (page 156)

LUNCH (FAST FUEL)

Salmon Soba Noodle Bowl (page 36)

DINNER (FAST FUEL)

Chicken Schnitzel (page 67)

SNACK 1 (SLOW FUEL)

1/2 chicken breast
Raw cut-up slow-fuel veggies

SNACK 2 (FAST FUEL)

Just Beet It Juice (page 175)

DAY 11

BREAKFAST (FAST FUEL)

Scrambled eggs (3–4 for men, 2 for women)
Red Grapefruit Juice (page 176)

LUNCH (FAST FUEL)

Guilt-Free Sloppy Joe (page 49)

DINNER (FAST FUEL)

Giant scallops (6–8 ounces for men, 3–5
 ounces for women) sautéed in 1 tablespoon
 olive oil
Stewed tomatoes
Brown rice, cooked (1 cup for men, 1/2 cup
 for women)

SNACK 1 (SLOW FUEL)

Cucumber Tuna Boats (page 151)

SNACK 2 (FAST FUEL)

**Strawberry and Pineapple Smoothie
 (page 162)**

DAY 12

BREAKFAST (FAST FUEL)

Tropical Açai Bowl (page 33)

LUNCH (FAST FUEL)

Chicken Coleslaw Salad (page 37)

DINNER (FAST FUEL)

Ginger Beef (page 83)

SNACK 1 (SLOW FUEL)

Cucumber Tuna Boats (page 151)

SNACK 2 (FAST FUEL)

Blended Super Juice (page 172)

DAY 13

BREAKFAST (FAST FUEL)

Sunrise Egg Muffin (page 30)

LUNCH (FAST FUEL)

Leftover Chicken Coleslaw Salad (page 37)

DINNER (FAST FUEL)

Slow Cooker Indian Lamb Curry (page 85)

SNACK 1 (SLOW FUEL)

Almond Delight Smoothie (page 169)

SNACK 2 (FAST FUEL)

Banana Blueberry Cookies (page 184)

DAY 14

BREAKFAST (FAST FUEL)

Scrambled eggs (3-4 for men, 2 for women)
Raspberry Tang Juice (page 178)

LUNCH (FAST FUEL)

Leftover **Slow Cooker Indian Lamb Curry
(page 85)**

DINNER (FAST FUEL)

Coriander Baked Salmon (page 60)

SNACK 1 (SLOW FUEL)

2-3 ounces tuna
1 cup kale chips

SNACK 2 (FAST FUEL)

**No-Bake Chocolate Apple Oatmeal Cookies
(page 182)**

VEGETABLES

1 bunch celery

1 red onion

1 white onion

One 12-ounce package frozen Asian vegetables

2 bags baby spinach

1 bag prewashed lettuce

1 bag fresh shredded kale

1–2 bags fresh spinach

1 large head red cabbage

2 cucumbers

4 English cucumbers

1 package carrots

2 red bell peppers

1 package fresh dill

1 package baby arugula

1 package collard greens

2 cups fresh green beans

1 package fresh sage

1 bunch cilantro

1 tomato

1 package cherry tomatoes

One 14.5-ounce can diced tomatoes

2 cups fingerling potatoes

2–3 beets

1 bunch asparagus

1 bunch scallions

1 red or green chile

1 small can 100 percent pure pumpkin puree

One 15-ounce can stewed tomatoes

FRUITS

1 lemon

1 bag frozen blueberries

1 bag frozen strawberries

1 bag frozen pineapple chunks

1 large carton fresh strawberries

1 large carton fresh raspberries

1 small carton fresh blueberries

2–3 avocados

6 bananas

1 small bottle orange juice

1 small bottle pineapple juice

5 apples

2 grapefruits

1 orange

1 small can pineapple chunks in juice

1 bag dried figs

1 bag dried blueberries

1 bag dried apples

5 dates, pitted

POULTRY

Rotisserie chicken

Six 6-ounce skinless, boneless chicken breasts

11/2 pounds ground turkey

SEAFOOD

Four 6-ounce wild sea bass fillets

One 4-ounce salmon fillet

Six 3-ounce salmon fillets

2 pounds giant scallops

Four 5-ounce cans chunk light tuna packed in
water

MEATS

16 ounces tri-tip or sirloin steak

2 pounds lamb

4 pork loin chops

EGGS AND DAIRY

2 dozen eggs

1 package goat cheese

One 16-ounce carton plain low-fat Greek yogurt

1 carton unsweetened vanilla almond milk

1 carton unsweetened coconut milk

BREADS, CEREALS, PASTA, AND GRAINS

1 box packaged cereal such as Special K or a
high-fiber cereal such as raisin bran or Fiber
One

4 whole-grain flatbreads

8 large brown rice cakes

1 package soba (buckwheat) noodles

1 canister bread crumbs

1 small package granola

1–2 packages brown rice

1 package wild rice

1 loaf whole-wheat bread

6 hamburger buns

NUTS AND SEEDS

1 package pumpkin seeds

1 package sunflower seeds

1 package flaxseed

MISCELLANEOUS

1 jar almond butter

1 bottle sesame oil

One 8-ounce package unsweetened frozen açai
puree

1 large can tomato sauce

1 small can tomato paste

1 small box cornstarch

BLOCK 3 WEEK 3 SAMPLE MENU (4 FAST FUELS DAILY)

DAY 15

BREAKFAST (FAST FUEL)

Baked Potatoes with Eggs (page 29)

LUNCH (FAST FUEL)

Pesto Steak Sandwich (page 54)

DINNER (FAST FUEL)

Turkey Picadillo (page 78)

SNACK 1 (SLOW FUEL)

Crabmeat-Stuffed Avocado (page 149)

SNACK 2 (FAST FUEL)

Pineapple Power Smoothie (page 159)

DAY 16

BREAKFAST (FAST FUEL)

Broccoli and Goat Cheese Omelet with Toast (page 31)

LUNCH (FAST FUEL)

Leftover **Turkey Picadillo (page 78)**

DINNER (FAST FUEL)

Dinner out: Sushi
Seaweed salad

SNACK 1 (SLOW FUEL)

½ grilled chicken breast
8 ounces **Fuelin' Veggie Juice 2 (page 174)**

SNACK 2 (FAST FUEL)

Green Zen Smoothie (page 164)

DAY 17

BREAKFAST (FAST FUEL)

Complete Morning Glory (page 26)

LUNCH (FAST FUEL)

Salmon Salad Sandwich (page 35)

DINNER (FAST FUEL)

Ginger Beef (page 83)

SNACK 1 (SLOW FUEL)

½ chicken breast
Raw cut-up slow-fuel veggies

SNACK 2 (FAST FUEL)

Sliced cucumbers dipped in hummus (1 cup
  for men, ½ cup for women)

DAY 18

BREAKFAST (FAST FUEL)

Baked Egg in a Hole (page 25)

LUNCH (FAST FUEL)

Leftover **Ginger Beef (page 83)** or Leftover
  Salmon Salad Sandwich (page 35)

DINNER (FAST FUEL)

Rotisserie chicken, skin removed (6–8 ounces
  for men, 3–5 ounces for women)
Shredded fresh cabbage dressed with
  1 tablespoon low-fat mayonnaise and
  2 tablespoons freshly squeezed lemon juice
**Chocolate Strawberry Chia Pudding
  (page 187)**

SNACK 1 (FAST FUEL)

Apple Melontini Smoothie (page 166)

SNACK 2 (SLOW FUEL)

Stuffed Eggs (page 150)

DAY 19

BREAKFAST (FAST FUEL)

Hard-boiled eggs (3–4 for men, 2 for women)
Watermelon Basil Juice (page 179)

LUNCH (FAST FUEL)

Leftover rotisserie chicken (6–8 ounces for
men, 3–5 ounces for women)
Raw broccoli and cauliflower florets
Leftover **Chocolate Strawberry Chia Pudding
(page 187)**

DINNER (SLOW FUEL)

2 grilled or broiled lamb chops (6–8 ounces
for men, 3–5 ounces for women)
Roasted red bell peppers

SNACK 1 (FAST FUEL)

Mango Ginger Smoothie (page 167)

SNACK 2 (FAST FUEL)

No-Bake Almond Butter Squares (page 183)

DAY 20

BREAKFAST (FAST FUEL)

Canadian bacon (4 slices for men, 2 slices
for women)
1¼ cups packaged cereal such as Special K
or a high-fiber cereal such as raisin bran or
Fiber One
1 cup almond milk

LUNCH (FAST FUEL)

Chicken Orzo Salad (page 38)

DINNER (FAST FUEL)

Baked tilapia seasoned with lemon pepper
Roasted Brussels sprouts (coat with olive oil
cooking spray and sprinkle with garlic salt
prior to roasting)
Strawberry Frozen Yogurt (page 193)

SNACK 1 (SLOW FUEL)

Almond Delight Smoothie (page 169)

SNACK 2 (FAST FUEL)

Zucchini Fries (page 93)

DAY 21

BREAKFAST (FAST FUEL)

Baked Potatoes with Eggs (page 29)

LUNCH (FAST FUEL)

Leftover tilapia and **Zucchini Fries (page 93)**

DINNER (FAST FUEL)

Sirloin steak (6–8 ounces for men, 3–5 ounces
  for women)
Tossed salad with 1–2 tablespoons low-fat
  salad dressing
Strawberry Frozen Yogurt (page 193)

SNACK 1 (SLOW FUEL)

2–3 ounces tuna
1 cup kale chips

SNACK 2 (FAST FUEL)

Peach Pie Smoothie (page 163)

VEGETABLES

1 bunch celery

1–2 red onions

2 white onions

1 large yellow onion

1 bunch scallions

1 small head butter lettuce

1 small head cabbage

Fresh ginger

One 12-ounce package frozen Asian vegetables

1 bunch scallions

1 bunch fresh parsley

1 bag fresh spinach

1 bag frozen spinach

1 bag mixed greens (for salads)

1 bag baby carrots

3–4 cucumbers

1 English cucumber

1 package carrots

1 bottle tomato juice

2 red bell peppers

1 green bell pepper

1 package fresh dill

2 packages baby arugula

1 package fresh mint

1 bunch cilantro

4 tomatoes

1–2 heads broccoli

1 package raw broccoli and cauliflower florets

1 package Brussels sprouts

4 zucchini

12 medium russet potatoes

1 package fresh basil

FRUITS

1 lime

1 bag frozen mango

1 bag frozen peaches

2 bags frozen strawberries

1 small carton fresh strawberries

1 small carton fresh blueberries

6 avocados

1 banana

1 bag frozen pineapple chunks

1 small bottle pineapple juice

1 small bag raisins

2 apples

1 cantaloupe

1 package seedless watermelon chunks

POULTRY

1 rotisserie chicken

1 pound ground turkey

1 package turkey links

1 package turkey bacon

SEAFOOD

Two 4-ounce cans salmon packed in water
Three 5-ounce cans tuna packed in water

6 ounces crabmeat
1 package tilapia fillets

MEATS

2 pounds London broil
1–2 sirloin steaks
1 package Canadian bacon

1 package turkey bacon
16 ounces tri-tip or sirloin steak

EGGS AND DAIRY

21/2 dozen eggs
1 package shredded reduced-fat sharp cheddar
  cheese

One 16-ounce carton plain low-fat Greek yogurt
1 carton unsweetened almond milk

BREADS, CEREALS, PASTA, AND GRAINS

Several packages brown rice

1 loaf whole-wheat bread

MISCELLANEOUS

1 bottle low-fat salad dressing
One 8-ounce can tomato sauce
1 jar green olives
1 jar capers
1 jar roasted red peppers
1 jar pesto sauce

1 jar Montreal steak seasoning
1 package kale chips
1 carton plain hummus
1 carton panko (Japanese-style bread crumbs)
1 small bottle white wine

SAMPLE BLOCK 2 MENUS

MEAL DESIGN FOR BLOCK 2

Breakfast Pattern: protein + 1 fast-fuel carb
Lunch Pattern: protein + 1 fast-fuel carb + slow-fuel carbs
Dinner Pattern: protein + slow-fuel carbs
Snack Pattern (1 midmorning, 1 midafternoon): Protein + nuts or seeds or a slow-fuel carb (or, after a workout, protein + a fast-fuel carb, if not eaten at one of your three main meals)

Stay on Block 2 for 2 weeks.

BLOCK 2 WEEK 1 SAMPLE MENU (2 FAST FUELS DAILY)

DAY 1

BREAKFAST (FAST FUEL)

Canadian bacon (4 slices for men, 2 slices for women), pan-fried

11/4 cups packaged cereal such as Special K or a high-fiber cereal like raisin bran or Fiber One

1 cup almond milk for the cereal

LUNCH (FAST FUEL)

Salmon Soba Noodle Bowl (page 36)

DINNER (SLOW FUEL)

Asian Ginger Chicken (page 126)

SNACK 1 (SLOW FUEL)

Celery spread with almond butter

SNACK 2 (SLOW FUEL)

1 hard-boiled egg
Handful of almonds

DAY 2

BREAKFAST (FAST FUEL)

Sunrise Smoothie (page 156)

LUNCH (FAST FUEL)

Chicken Kale Soup (page 45)

DINNER (SLOW FUEL)

Ham Pesto Zoodles (page 141)

SNACK 1 (SLOW FUEL)

1 hard-boiled egg
Handful of almonds

SNACK 2 (SLOW FUEL)

1/2 grilled chicken breast
8 ounces **Fuelin' Veggie Juice 2 (page 174)**

DAY 3

BREAKFAST (SLOW FUEL)

Egg and Squash Skillet (page 100)

LUNCH (FAST FUEL)

Hawaiian BBQ Chicken Pizza (page 42) or
Leftover **Chicken Kale Soup (page 45)**

DINNER (SLOW FUEL)

**Blackened Grouper and Snap Peas
(page 130)**

SNACK 1 (FAST FUEL)

Sunshine Sorbet (page 194)

SNACK 2 (SLOW FUEL)

Cucumber Tuna Boats (page 151)

DAY 4

BREAKFAST (FAST FUEL)

**Broccoli and Goat Cheese Omelet with Toast
(page 31)**

LUNCH (FAST FUEL)

Southwestern Orzo Salad (page 52)

DINNER (SLOW FUEL)

Tri-Tip and Broccolini (page 138)

SNACK 1 (SLOW FUEL)

Leftover **Cucumber Tuna Boats (page 151)**

SNACK 2 (SLOW FUEL)

Almond Delight Smoothie (page 169)

DAY 5

BREAKFAST (SLOW FUEL)

Eggs in a Nest (page 101)

LUNCH (SLOW FUEL)

Grilled Shrimp and Spinach Salad (page 114)

DINNER (FAST FUEL)

Low-Fat Lasagna (page 79)

SNACK 1 (FAST FUEL)

Protein Carrot Cake Bites (page 188)

SNACK 2 (SLOW FUEL)

2–3 ounces tuna
1 cup kale chips

DAY 6

BREAKFAST (SLOW FUEL)

Bacon Scrambled over Asparagus (page 102)

LUNCH (FAST FUEL)

Salmon Salad Sandwich (page 35)

DINNER (SLOW FUEL)

Restaurant dinner, with grilled steak
Steamed side vegetables
Tossed salad with oil and vinegar dressing

SNACK 1 (FAST FUEL)

Quinoa and Turkey Chorizo–Stuffed Chiles (page 90)

SNACK 2 (SLOW FUEL)

1 hard-boiled egg
Handful of almonds

DAY 7

BREAKFAST (SLOW FUEL)

Athletic Omelet (page 105)

LUNCH (FAST FUEL)

Chicken and White Bean Soup (page 46)

DINNER (SLOW FUEL)

Roast turkey breast (6–8 ounces for men, 3–5
  ounces for women)
Steamed cauliflower
Tossed salad with 1–2 tablespoons low-fat
  salad dressing

SNACK 1 (SLOW FUEL)

2–3 ounces leftover roast turkey breast
8 ounces **Fuelin' Veggie Juice 2 (page 174)**

SNACK 2 (FAST FUEL)

Leftover **Quinoa and Turkey Chorizo–Stuffed
  Chiles (page 90)**

VEGETABLES

1 bunch celery
2 red onions
2–3 white onions
1 small head butter lettuce
1 bunch scallions
4 bags fresh spinach
4 bags baby spinach
1 bag fresh kale
1 bag mixed greens (for salads)
3–4 cucumbers
4 English cucumbers
1 package carrots
1 bottle tomato juice
1–2 red bell peppers
1–2 green bell peppers
4 large poblano chiles
1 red jalapeño
1 green jalapeño
1 package fresh dill
1 package fresh basil
1 package fresh chives

2 bunches cilantro
1 bunch parsley
2 tomatoes
2 heirloom tomatoes
3 cups snap peas
1 package cherry tomatoes
1 bunch broccoli
1 large bunch broccolini
1 large package button mushrooms
2 portobello mushroom caps
1 large package shiitake mushrooms
5 to 6 medium zucchini
6 summer squash
One 15-ounce can black beans
One 15-ounce can corn
6 small Yukon Gold potatoes
1 package fresh rosemary
1 package fresh thyme
2 bunches asparagus
1 bag frozen cauliflower
Two 15-ounce cans cannellini beans

FRUITS

1 bag frozen blueberries
1 bag frozen mango
2 avocados
3 bananas

1 small bottle orange juice
1 small can pineapple chunks in juice
6 dates

POULTRY

1–2 rotisserie chickens
2 skinless, boneless chicken breasts
One 12-ounce can chicken breast packed in
  water

1 pound ground turkey
12 ounces turkey chorizo
1 turkey breast

SEAFOOD

One 4-ounce salmon fillet

Four 4-ounce grouper fillets

Four 5-ounce cans chunk light tuna packed in water

2 pounds large shrimp

One 3-ounce can tuna packed in water

Two 4-ounce cans salmon packed in water

MEATS

1 package Canadian bacon

1 small package ham

16 ounces tri-tip

EGGS AND DAIRY

21/2 dozen eggs

1 large package shredded reduced-fat mozzarella

16 ounces part-skim ricotta

1 package queso fresco

1 carton grated Parmesan cheese

1 package goat cheese

1 package shredded reduced-fat cheddar cheese

1 carton unsweetened almond milk

BREADS, CEREALS, PASTA, AND GRAINS

1 package cereal such as Special K or a high-fiber cereal such as raisin bran or Fiber One

1 package soba noodles

1 package kelp noodles

4 whole-wheat tortillas

1 pound lasagna noodles

1 package whole-wheat orzo

1 loaf whole-wheat bread

NUTS AND SEEDS

Several packages raw almonds

1 package unsweetened shredded coconut

MISCELLANEOUS

Five 14.5-ounce cans low-sodium, low-fat chicken broth

1 bottle barbecue sauce

1 package kale chips

One 46-ounce jar low-sugar or low-carbohydrate pasta sauce

1 stick butter

BLOCK 2 WEEK 2 SAMPLE MENU (2 FAST FUELS DAILY)

DAY 8

BREAKFAST (FAST FUEL)

Breakfast Cups (page 99)
1/2 grapefruit

LUNCH (SLOW FUEL)

Shrimp Salad Wraps (page 117)

DINNER (SLOW FUEL)

2 grilled or broiled pork chops (6–8 ounces
  for men, 3–5 ounces for women) with
  teriyaki sauce
Steamed yellow squash
Steamed spinach

SNACK 1 (FAST FUEL)

**No-Bake Almond Butter Banana Bites
  (page 190)**

SNACK 2 (SLOW FUEL)

1 hard-boiled egg
Handful of almonds

DAY 9

BREAKFAST (SLOW FUEL)

**Smoked Ham and Spinach Quiche
  (page 106)**

LUNCH (FAST FUEL)

Taco Lettuce Boats (page 123)
1 apple

DINNER (SLOW FUEL)

Asian takeout of mixed steamed vegetables
  and shrimp (2 cups for men, 1 cup for
  women)

SNACK 1 (FAST FUEL)

Pineapple Power Smoothie (page 159)

SNACK 2 (SLOW FUEL)

Stuffed Eggs (page 150)

DAY 10

BREAKFAST (FAST FUEL)

Smoked Gouda and Veggie Frittata (page 104)
1/2 grapefruit

LUNCH (SLOW FUEL)

Vietnamese Chicken Salad (page 118)

DINNER (SLOW FUEL)

Ham Pesto Zoodles (page 141)

SNACK 1 (FAST FUEL)

The Hulk Smoothie (page 165)

SNACK 2 (SLOW FUEL)

Leftover **Stuffed Eggs (page 150)**

DAY 11

BREAKFAST (FAST FUEL)

Athletic Omelet (page 105)
1 peach

LUNCH (FAST FUEL)

Sliced deli roast beef (6–8 ounces for men, 3–5 ounces for women) with 1 tablespoon mustard on rye bread (2 slices for men, 1 slice for women)
Dill pickle
Sliced tomato

DINNER (SLOW FUEL)

Rotisserie chicken, skin removed (6–8 ounces for men, 3–5 ounces for women)
Shredded fresh cabbage dressed with 1 tablespoon low-fat mayonnaise and 2 tablespoons lemon juice

SNACK 1 (SLOW FUEL)

Almond Delight Smoothie (page 169)

SNACK 2 (SLOW FUEL)

Leftover **Stuffed Eggs (page 150)**

DAY 12

BREAKFAST (FAST FUEL)

Sunrise Smoothie (page 156)

LUNCH (FAST FUEL)

Leftover rotisserie chicken (6–8 ounces for men, 3–5 ounces for women)
Raw broccoli and cauliflower florets
1 medium apple

DINNER (SLOW FUEL)

Filet Mignon Skewers (page 144)

SNACK 1 (SLOW FUEL)

2–3 ounces tuna
1 cup kale chips

SNACK 2 (SLOW FUEL)

Celery spread with almond butter

DAY 13

BREAKFAST (FAST FUEL)

Baked Potatoes with Eggs (page 29)

LUNCH (SLOW FUEL)

Leftover **Filet Mignon Skewers (page 144)**

DINNER (SLOW FUEL)

Baked tilapia (6–8 ounces for men, 3–5 ounces for women), seasoned with lemon pepper
Roasted Brussels sprouts (coat with olive oil cooking spray and sprinkle with garlic salt prior to roasting)
Tossed salad with 1–2 tablespoons low-fat salad dressing

SNACK 1 (FAST FUEL)

Strawberry Frozen Yogurt (page 193)

SNACK 2 (SLOW FUEL)

1/2 grilled chicken breast or 2–3 ounces leftover tilapia
8 ounces **Fuelin' Veggie Juice 2 (page 174)**

DAY 14

BREAKFAST (FAST FUEL)

Sunrise Egg Muffin (page 30)

LUNCH (SLOW FUEL)

Spicy Shrimp Cobb Salad (page 115)

DINNER (FAST FUEL)

Grilled sirloin steak (6 ounces for men,
  4 ounces for women)
Steamed cauliflower
Tossed salad with 1–2 tablespoons low-fat
  salad dressing
Leftover **Strawberry Frozen Yogurt
  (page 193)**

SNACK 1 (SLOW FUEL)

1 hard-boiled egg
Handful of almonds

SNACK 2 (SLOW FUEL)

1/2 chicken breast
Assorted raw cut-up slow-fuel veggies

VEGETABLES

1 bunch celery

2 red onions

1 white onion

1 small head Boston lettuce

1 head cabbage

1 bunch scallions

7 shallots

1 bag fresh spinach

4 bags baby spinach

1 bag mixed greens (for salads)

1 package romaine salad

1 bag baby carrots

2 cucumbers

1 package carrots

1 bottle tomato juice

1–2 red bell peppers

1–2 green bell peppers

1 package fresh mint

1 package fresh basil

2 bunches cilantro

3 tomatoes

2 heirloom tomatoes

1 package grape tomatoes

1 package cherry tomatoes

1 bunch broccoli

1 package broccoli and cauliflower florets

1 package Brussels sprouts

1–2 small cans sliced button mushrooms

1 package fresh sliced mushrooms

3 portobello mushroom caps

8 medium zucchini

2–3 yellow summer squash

One 15-ounce can corn

6 Idaho potatoes

1 bag frozen spinach

1 small package frozen peas

1 bag frozen cauliflower

FRUITS

1 grapefruit

2 apples

1 peach

1 green apple

1 green pear

1 kiwi

1 bag frozen pineapple chunks

1 bag frozen strawberries

1 bag frozen blueberries

1 small carton fresh strawberries

2 avocados

5 bananas

1 small bottle orange juice

1 small bottle pineapple juice

POULTRY

1 package smoked turkey ham

1 whole chicken

1–2 rotisserie chickens

1 package turkey bacon

SEAFOOD

2 pounds cooked shrimp

Two 5-ounce cans tuna packed in water

One 3-ounce can tuna packed in water

1 package tilapia fillets

MEATS

2 pork chops

1 package Canadian bacon

1 small package ham

1/2 pound deli roast beef

11/2 pounds lean filet mignon

Sirloin steak

EGGS AND DAIRY

4 dozen eggs

1 small package shredded Swiss cheese

1 package smoked Gouda

1 package low-fat shredded cheddar cheese

1 small carton fat-free cottage cheese

1 small carton milk

1 carton unsweetened almond milk

BREADS, CEREALS, PASTA, AND GRAINS

1 loaf rye bread

1 package whole-wheat English muffins

MISCELLANEOUS

1 package dark chocolate chips

1 jar almond butter

1 jar dill pickles

1 small package crackers

SAMPLE BLOCK 1 MENUS

MEAL DESIGN FOR BLOCK 1

Breakfast Pattern: protein + 1 fast-fuel carb or 1 slow-fuel carb

Lunch Pattern: protein + slow-fuel carb

Dinner Pattern: protein + slow-fuel carb

Snack Pattern (1 midmorning, 1 midafternoon): protein + nuts or seeds or a slow-fuel carb (or, after a workout, protein + a slow-fuel carb, if not eaten at one of your three main meals)

Stay on Block 1 for only 1 week.

BLOCK 1 ONE-WEEK SAMPLE MENU (1 FAST FUEL DAILY)

DAY 1

BREAKFAST (FAST FUEL)

Baked Egg in a Hole (page 25)

LUNCH (SLOW FUEL)

Corn Chowder with Shrimp and Bacon
(page 111)

DINNER (SLOW FUEL)

Chicken Zoodles Chow Mein (page 128)

SNACK 1 (SLOW FUEL)

Stuffed Eggs (page 150)

SNACK 2 (SLOW FUEL)

Almond Delight Smoothie (page 169)

DAY 2

BREAKFAST (FAST FUEL)

Turkey sausage links or patties (4 pieces for
    men, 2 pieces for women), pan-fried
Whole-grain or sprouted-grain toast (2 slices
    for men, 1 slice for women), with all-fruit jam
    if desired

LUNCH (SLOW FUEL)

Refreshing Cucumber Salad with Tuna
(page 108)

DINNER (SLOW FUEL)

Herbed Chicken Breasts (page 137)

SNACK 1 (SLOW FUEL)

Leftover **Stuffed Eggs (page 150)**

SNACK 2 (SLOW FUEL)

1/2 grilled chicken breast
8 ounces **Fuelin' Veggie Juice 2 (page 174)**

DAY 3

BREAKFAST (FAST FUEL)

Sunrise Smoothie (page 156)

LUNCH (SLOW FUEL)

Turkey Lettuce Wraps (page 122)

DINNER (SLOW FUEL)

Cauliflower Casserole (page 148)

SNACK 1 (SLOW FUEL)

1 hard-boiled egg
Handful of almonds

SNACK 2 (SLOW FUEL)

Cucumber Tuna Boats (page 151)

DAY 4

BREAKFAST (SLOW FUEL)

**Baked Broccoli and Cheddar Frittata
   (page 103)**

LUNCH (SLOW FUEL)

Zucchini and Salmon Salad (page 112)

DINNER (SLOW FUEL)

**Chicken Parmesan with Spaghetti Squash
   (page 134)**

SNACK 1 (SLOW FUEL)

Leftover **Stuffed Eggs (page 150)**

SNACK 2 (FAST FUEL)

Sunshine Sorbet (page 194)

DAY 5

BREAKFAST (SLOW FUEL)

Athletic Omelet (page 105)

LUNCH (SLOW FUEL)

Salad bar: 1–2 cups fresh greens, 1/2 cup kidney beans or chickpeas, tomato slices, chopped green bell peppers, 1 tablespoon sunflower seeds, 1–2 tablespoons low-fat salad dressing

DINNER (SLOW FUEL)

Leftover **Chicken Parmesan with Spaghetti Squash (page 134)**

SNACK 1 (SLOW FUEL)

2–3 ounces leftover chicken
Assorted raw cut-up slow-fuel veggies (such as carrots, cauliflower, broccoli, celery, or bell peppers)

SNACK 2 (FAST FUEL)

Almond Delight Smoothie (page 169)

DAY 6

BREAKFAST (SLOW FUEL)

Breakfast Cups (page 99)

LUNCH (SLOW FUEL)

Garlic Chicken Broccolini Salad (page 119)

DINNER (SLOW FUEL)

Asian takeout of mixed steamed vegetables and shrimp (2 cups for men, 1 cup for women)

SNACK 1 (FAST FUEL)

Mango Ginger Smoothie (page 167)

SNACK 2 (SLOW FUEL)

1 hard-boiled egg
Handful of almonds

DAY 7

BREAKFAST (SLOW FUEL)

Eggs in a Nest (page 101)

LUNCH (SLOW FUEL)

Turkey Lettuce Wraps (page 122)

DINNER (FAST FUEL)

Easy Linguine with Meat Sauce (page 84)

SNACK 1 (SLOW FUEL)

Almond Delight Smoothie (page 169)

SNACK 2 (SLOW FUEL)

1 hard-boiled egg
Handful of almonds

VEGETABLES

1 bunch celery

4–5 onions

1 head lettuce

Fresh ginger

1 package garlic cloves

1 bunch of green onions

1 bunch of scallions

6 large shallots

1 bag fresh spinach

1 bag baby spinach

1 bag baby carrots

2 cucumbers

5–6 Persian cucumbers

2 English cucumbers

1 package carrots

1–2 red bell peppers

2–3 green bell peppers

2 packages fresh dill

1 package fresh oregano

1 package fresh basil

1 package fresh chives

2 bunches cilantro

1 bunch parsley

1 tomato

2 packages grape tomatoes

1 package cherry tomatoes

One 14.5-ounce can diced tomatoes

1 bunch broccoli

1 large head cauliflower

1 spaghetti squash

1 package broccoli and cauliflower florets

2 pounds string beans

11/2 pounds broccolini

1 cup sliced button mushrooms

2 portobello mushroom caps

4 medium zucchini

Three 15-ounce cans corn

1 package fresh thyme

FRUITS

1 lemon

1 bag frozen pineapple chunks

1 bag frozen blueberries

1 bag frozen mangoes

2 avocados

2 bananas

1 small bottle orange juice

1 fresh mango

POULTRY

1 pound ground chicken breast

8 skinless, boneless chicken breasts

12 slices deli turkey

1 rotisserie chicken

1 package turkey links, sausage flavored

SEAFOOD

3/4 pound peeled and deveined medium shrimp

Four 5-ounce cans tuna packed in water

Four 2-ounce salmon fillets

MEATS

1 package bacon

1 package Canadian bacon

1/2 pound lean ground beef

EGGS AND DAIRY

31/2 dozen eggs

1 small package shredded Swiss cheese

1 package fat-free shredded mozzarella

1 carton grated Parmesan cheese

1 package feta cheese

1 large package shredded reduced-fat cheddar
  cheese

1 small chunk Parmigiano-Reggiano cheese

One 16-ounce carton plain low-fat Greek yogurt

1 small carton low-fat milk

1 carton unsweetened almond milk

1 small container half-and-half

BREADS, CEREALS, PASTA, AND GRAINS

1 box whole-wheat linguine

1 loaf whole-wheat bread

NUTS AND SEEDS

1 small jar sesame seeds

1 small package pine nuts

MISCELLANEOUS

Two 14.5-ounce cans low-sodium, low-fat
  chicken broth

1 small can tomato paste

One 46-ounce jar of low-sugar or low-
  carbohydrate pasta sauce

Can you calorie-cycle your way to a leaner physique and better muscle definition if you're vegan or vegetarian? You bet! A plant-based diet is an excellent way to eat. Plus, as long as the world is populated with vegans and vegetarians, well, that's more rib-eyes for me.

There are various types of "plant eaters," from vegans who eat no animal products whatsoever to folks who don't eat chicken or beef but might enjoy some fish now and then (sometimes called pescatarians). If you're in the vegan crowd, your diet consists of soy foods, beans and legumes, grains, fruits, vegetables, nuts, and seeds. You get your protein from soy, beans, legumes, nuts, and seeds. It's best for you to focus on beans and legumes as your chief sources of protein, since nuts are high in calories for such little packages. You'd probably pack on pounds if you ate too many nuts.

Some notes for vegetarians:

Semi-vegetarian: You eat dairy, eggs, poultry, and fish but avoid red meat. If you're in this category, the menus in the previous section will work for you easily. You'll want to try to eat more poultry and fish, and because you have no problem with eggs, eat more of those, too. So where I call for red meat, pork, veal, or lamb, simply substitute any of the other proteins, such as poultry or fish.

Lacto-ovo-vegetarian: You eat eggs and dairy products but avoid poultry, fish, and red meat. While following my menus, you can include eggs, dairy foods, and non-dairy milks as a protein source, but you'll get most of your other protein from beans, legumes, nuts, and seeds. My plan includes a tiny bit of dairy, as well as non-dairy milks.

Lacto-vegetarian: You eat dairy but avoid all other animal products and eggs. To follow my plan, you can enjoy the vegan recipes, supported by dairy foods you enjoy.

In the section below, I'm giving you sample menus for fully plant-based calorie-cycling meals. You'll find a one-week sample for Block 3, a one-week sample for Block 2, and a one-week sample for Block 1.

PLANT-BASED: BLOCK 3 SAMPLE MENU
(4 FAST FUELS DAILY)

DAY 1

BREAKFAST (FAST FUEL)

11/4 cups packaged cereal such as Special K
   or a high-fiber cereal such as raisin bran or
   Fiber One
1 tablespoon hemp seeds to sprinkle over
   your cereal
1 cup almond milk

LUNCH (FAST FUEL)

Tofu Orzo Bowl (page 57)

DINNER (FAST FUEL)

1 or 2 portobello mushrooms, sautéed in
   1 tablespoon olive oil
Steamed asparagus
1 baked potato, topped with 1–2 tablespoons
   dairy-free sour cream if desired

SNACK 1 (FAST FUEL)

Green Zen Smoothie (page 164)

SNACK 2 (SLOW FUEL)

Baby carrots and other raw veggies

DAY 2

BREAKFAST (FAST FUEL)

Tropical Açai Bowl (page 33)

LUNCH (FAST FUEL)

Vegetable wraps: alfalfa sprouts, cucumber
   slices, tomato slices, and 2 slices avocado in
   a whole-wheat tortilla spread with 2–3
   tablespoons hummus

DINNER (FAST FUEL)

Pinto beans (1 cup for men, 1/2 cup for
   women)
Kale sautéed in 1 tablespoon olive oil
Brown rice, cooked (1 cup for men, 1/2 cup
   for women)

SNACK 1 (SLOW FUEL)

Handful of almonds
8 ounces **Fuelin' Veggie Juice 2 (page 174)**

SNACK 2 (FAST FUEL)

Blueberry Dream Smoothie (page 157)

DAY 3

BREAKFAST (SLOW FUEL)

Almond Delight Smoothie (page 169)

LUNCH (FAST FUEL)

Chicken and White Bean Soup (page 46)
(replace the chicken in the recipe with an additional 1/2 to 1 cup canned white beans and use low-sodium, low fat vegetable broth)

DINNER (FAST FUEL)

Garbanzo beans (1 cup for men, 1/2 cup for women) on a bed of mixed salad greens, drizzled with low-fat salad dressing
Whole-grain or sprouted-grain bread (2 slices for men, 1 slice for women)

SNACK 1 (SLOW FUEL)

Handful of almonds
Raw cut-up slow-fuel veggies

SNACK 2 (FAST FUEL)

Strawberry and Pineapple Smoothie (page 162)

DAY 4

BREAKFAST (FAST FUEL)

Cooked quinoa (1 cup for men, 1/2 cup for women), sweetened with a little cinnamon and honey
1/2 grapefruit

LUNCH (FAST FUEL)

Mixed greens and salad vegetables topped with cubed tofu (1 cup for men, 1/2 cup for women) and drizzled with 1 tablespoon olive oil and 1 tablespoon balsamic vinegar
1 apple

DINNER (FAST FUEL)

Veggie Enchiladas (page 89) (use a non-dairy shredded cheese in place of the Mexican cheese)

SNACK 1 (SLOW FUEL)

Handful of almonds
Assorted chopped raw vegetables

SNACK 2 (FAST FUEL)

Almond Butter and Jelly Rice Cakes (page 96)

DAY 5

BREAKFAST (FAST FUEL)

Green with Envy Juice (page 170)

LUNCH (SLOW FUEL)

Vegan Lentil Salad (page 107)

DINNER (FAST FUEL)

Light Meatless Spaghetti (page 88) (omit
   the half-and-half)

SNACK 1 (FAST FUEL)

Handful of almonds
1 peach or other seasonal fruit

SNACK 2 (FAST FUEL)

Sunshine Sorbet (page 194)

DAY 6

BREAKFAST (FAST FUEL)

1 cup non-dairy yogurt
1 cup fresh berries

LUNCH (FAST FUEL)

Leftover **Light Meatless Spaghetti (page 88)**

DINNER (FAST FUEL)

1 cup chopped cooked portobello
   mushrooms mixed with no-sugar-added
   pasta sauce and served over cooked whole-
   wheat pasta (1 cup for men, 1/2 cup for
   women)

SNACK 1 (SLOW FUEL)

Sliced cucumbers dipped in hummus (1 cup
   for men, 1/2 cup for women)

SNACK 2 (FAST FUEL)

Banana Blueberry Cookies (page 184)

DAY 7

BREAKFAST (FAST FUEL)

2 veggie sausage patties, pan-fried
1 tomato, sliced
Grits, cooked (1 cup for men, 1/2 cup for
  women)

LUNCH (FAST FUEL)

Organic lentil soup, canned (2 cups for men,
  1 cup for women)
Whole-grain or sprouted-grain bread (2 slices
  for men, 1 slice for women)

DINNER (FAST FUEL)

**Mushrooms, Tofu, and Baby Bok Choy
  (page 142)**
Sunshine Sorbet (page 194)

SNACK 1 (SLOW FUEL)

2 ounces non-dairy cheese
1 cup kale chips

SNACK 2 (FAST FUEL)

Leftover **Banana Blueberry Cookies
  (page 184)**

SHOPPING LIST FOR SAMPLE PLANT-BASED BLOCK 3: MAIN INGREDIENTS

VEGETABLES

1 package frozen stir-fry vegetables

1 package alfalfa sprouts

1 bunch celery

3 red onions

2–3 yellow onions

6 baby bok choy

Fresh ginger

1 bulb of garlic

1 bunch scallions

4 bags fresh spinach

1 bag fresh kale

1 bag mixed greens (for salads)

1 bag baby carrots

5–6 cucumbers

1 package carrots

2–3 red bell peppers

3–4 green bell peppers

2 packages fresh dill

1 package fresh basil

1 package fresh chives

1 bunch cilantro

3 tomatoes

1 package cherry tomatoes

1 package broccoli and cauliflower florets

1 large package button mushrooms

4 to 5 portobello mushroom caps

One 15-ounce can pinto beans

One 15-ounce can corn

1 russet potato

1 package fresh rosemary

1 package fresh thyme

1 bunch asparagus

1 bag frozen spinach

Four 15-ounce cans cannellini beans

One 15-ounce can garbanzo beans

One 15-ounce can black beans

One 15-ounce can plum tomatoes

1 package lentils

FRUITS

1 grapefruit

1 apple

2 green apples

1 peach

1 bag frozen pineapple chunks

1 bag frozen strawberries

1 bag frozen mango

1 small carton fresh strawberries

1 small carton fresh blueberries

1 avocado

7 bananas

5 dates

1 fresh mango

1 package dried blueberries

NON-DAIRY AND MEAT SUBSTITUTES

1–2 cartons unsweetened almond milk

2 cartons firm tofu

1 carton dairy-free sour cream

1 package non-dairy shredded cheese

1 block non-dairy cheese

1 large package imitation ground meat (textured vegetable protein)

One 8-ounce carton non-dairy yogurt

1 package veggie sausage patties

Two 15-ounce cans organic lentil soup

BREADS, CEREALS, PASTA, AND GRAINS

1 package cereal such as Special K or a high-fiber cereal such as raisin bran or Fiber One

1 package quinoa

8 large brown rice cakes

16 ounces whole-wheat pasta

1 package whole-wheat tortillas

1 package brown rice

1 package whole-wheat orzo

1 loaf whole-wheat bread

1 large carton oatmeal

1 large carton grits

NUTS AND SEEDS

Several packages raw almonds

1 package flaxseed

1 large package chia seeds

1 package hemp seeds

MISCELLANEOUS

1 bottle low-fat salad dressing

2 packages low-sodium, low-fat vegetable broth

One 15-ounce can enchilada sauce

1 small bottle white wine

1 jar almond butter

One 46-ounce jar low-sugar or low-carbohydrate pasta sauce

1 bottle lemon juice

1 bottle lime juice

1 bottle avocado oil

1 package kale chips

1 carton plain hummus

PLANT-BASED: BLOCK 2 SAMPLE MENU
(2 FAST FUELS DAILY)

DAY 1

BREAKFAST (FAST FUEL)

11/4 cups packaged cereal such as Special K
or a high-fiber cereal such as raisin bran or
Fiber One
1 tablespoon hemp seeds to sprinkle over
your cereal
1 cup almond milk

LUNCH (SLOW FUEL)

Organic vegetarian vegetable soup, canned
(2 cups for men, 1 cup for women)

DINNER (FAST FUEL)

Light Meatless Spaghetti (page 88)

SNACK 1 (SLOW FUEL)

Handful of almonds
Assorted raw slow-fuel vegetables

SNACK 2 (SLOW FUEL)

Almond Delight Smoothie (page 169)

DAY 2

BREAKFAST (FAST FUEL)

Blended Super Juice (page 172)

LUNCH (FAST FUEL)

Leftover **Light Meatless Spaghetti (page 88)**

DINNER (SLOW FUEL)

Vegan Slow Cooker Chili (page 145)

SNACK 1 (SLOW FUEL)

Handful of almonds
8 ounces **Fuelin' Veggie Juice 2 (page 174)**

SNACK 2 (SLOW FUEL)

Handful of pumpkin seeds
1 cup almond milk

DAY 3

BREAKFAST (FAST FUEL)

Tropical Açai Bowl (page 33)

LUNCH (SLOW FUEL)

Vegan Slow Cooker Chili (page 145)

DINNER (FAST FUEL)

Veggie Enchiladas (page 89) (use a non-dairy shredded cheese in place of the Mexican cheese)

SNACK 1 (SLOW FUEL)

Handful of almonds
Raw cut-up slow-fuel veggies

SNACK 2 (SLOW FUEL)

Almond Delight Smoothie (page 169)

DAY 4

BREAKFAST (FAST FUEL)

Cooked quinoa (1 cup for men, 1/2 cup for women), sweetened with a little cinnamon and honey
1/2 grapefruit

LUNCH (SLOW FUEL)

Vegan Lentil Salad (page 107)

DINNER (SLOW FUEL)

Veggie burger, pan-fried
Stewed tomatoes

SNACK 1 (SLOW FUEL)

Handful of almonds
Assorted chopped raw slow-fuel vegetables

SNACK 2 (FAST FUEL)

Green Zen Smoothie (page 164)

DAY 5

BREAKFAST (FAST FUEL)

Blueberry Dream Smoothie (page 157)

LUNCH (FAST FUEL)

Tofu Orzo Bowl (page 57)

DINNER (SLOW FUEL)

Mushrooms, Tofu, and Baby Bok Choy (page 142)

SNACK 1 (SLOW FUEL)

Handful of pumpkin seeds
1 cup almond milk

SNACK 2 (SLOW FUEL)

1 cup organic vegetarian vegetable soup, canned

DAY 6

BREAKFAST (FAST FUEL)

1 cup non-dairy yogurt
1 cup fresh berries

LUNCH (SLOW FUEL)

Leftover **Mushrooms, Tofu, and Baby Bok Choy (page 142)**

DINNER (FAST FUEL)

Light Meatless Spaghetti (page 88) (omit the half-and-half)

SNACK 1 (SLOW FUEL)

Almond Delight Smoothie (page 169)

SNACK 2 (SLOW FUEL)

Handful of almonds
Assorted raw cut-up slow-fuel vegetables

DAY 7

BREAKFAST (FAST FUEL)

2 veggie sausage patties, pan-fried
1 tomato, sliced
Grits, cooked (1 cup for men, 1/2 cup for
  women)

LUNCH (FAST FUEL)

Leftover **Light Meatless Spaghetti (page 88)**

DINNER (SLOW FUEL)

Vegan Slow Cooker Chili (page 145)

SNACK 1 (SLOW FUEL)

2 ounces non-dairy cheese
1 cup kale chips

SNACK 2 (SLOW FUEL)

8 ounces **Fuelin' Veggie Juice 2 (page 174)**

SHOPPING LIST FOR SAMPLE PLANT-BASED BLOCK 2: MAIN INGREDIENTS

VEGETABLES

1 bunch celery

3 red onions

3–4 yellow onions

6 baby bok choy

1 bunch scallions

1 bag fresh spinach

1 package collard greens

1 bag baby carrots

3 cucumbers

1 package carrots

1–2 red bell peppers

3–4 green bell peppers

2 packages fresh dill

1 package fresh mint

1 package fresh basil

2 bunches cilantro

1 tomato

Four 15-ounce cans diced tomatoes and green chiles

Three 28-ounce cans crushed tomatoes

1 package broccoli and cauliflower florets

1 large package button mushrooms

1 large portobello mushroom cap

One 15-ounce can corn

1 bunch parsley

1 bag frozen spinach

One 15-ounce can black beans

Two 15-ounce cans plum tomatoes

One 15-ounce can stewed tomatoes

1 bottle tomato juice

FRUITS

1 grapefruit

1 apple

1 bag frozen strawberries

1 bag frozen blueberries

1 bag frozen mango

1 small carton fresh strawberries

1 small carton fresh blueberries

1 avocado

3 bananas

1 small bottle pineapple juice

1 small can pineapple chunks in juice

NON-DAIRY AND MEAT SUBSTITUTES

1–2 cartons unsweetened almond milk

2 cartons firm tofu

2 large packages imitation ground meat (textured vegetable protein)

1 package veggie burgers

One 8-ounce carton non-dairy yogurt

Four 15-ounce cans vegetarian vegetable soup

BREADS, CEREALS, PASTA, AND GRAINS

2 boxes whole-wheat pasta

1 small package granola

1 package whole-wheat tortillas

NUTS AND SEEDS

1 package pumpkin seeds

MISCELLANEOUS

2 packages chili seasoning
One 8-ounce package unsweetened
  frozen açai puree
Two 15-ounce cans enchilada sauce
2 small bottles white wine
1 package kale chips

PLANT-BASED: BLOCK 1 SAMPLE MENU
(1 FAST FUEL DAILY)

DAY 1

BREAKFAST (FAST FUEL)

Tropical Açai Bowl (page 33)

LUNCH (SLOW FUEL)

Vegan Lentil Salad (page 107)

DINNER (SLOW FUEL)

1 or 2 portobello mushrooms, sautéed in
  1 tablespoon olive oil
Steamed asparagus

SNACK 1 (SLOW FUEL)

Handful of almonds
Assorted raw slow-fuel vegetables

SNACK 2 (SLOW FUEL)

Almond Delight Smoothie (page 169)

DAY 2

BREAKFAST (FAST FUEL)

**Strawberry and Pineapple Smoothie
(page 162)**

LUNCH (SLOW FUEL)

Vegetable wraps: alfalfa sprouts, cucumber
  slices, tomato slices, and 2 slices avocado
  wrapped in lettuce leaves with 2–3
  tablespoons hummus

DINNER (SLOW FUEL)

Faux chicken strips (1 cup for men, 1/2 cup
  for women) stir-fried with a package of
  frozen stir-fry vegetables, soy sauce, and
  1–2 tablespoons olive oil

SNACK 1 (SLOW FUEL)

Handful of almonds
8 ounces **Fuelin' Veggie Juice 2 (page 174)**

SNACK 2 (SLOW FUEL)

Handful of pumpkin seeds
1 cup almond milk

DAY 3

BREAKFAST (FAST FUEL)

Green Goddess Smoothie (page 173)

LUNCH (SLOW FUEL)

Vegan Lentil Salad (page 107)

DINNER (SLOW FUEL)

Garbanzo beans (1 cup for men, 1/2 cup for women) on a bed of mixed salad greens, drizzled with low-fat salad dressing

SNACK 1 (SLOW FUEL)

Handful of almonds
Raw cut-up slow-fuel veggies

SNACK 2 (SLOW FUEL)

Almond Delight Smoothie (page 169)

DAY 4

BREAKFAST (FAST FUEL)

Tropical Açai Bowl (page 33)

LUNCH (SLOW FUEL)

Mixed greens and salad vegetables topped with cubed tofu (1 cup for men, 1/2 cup for women), drizzled with 1 tablespoon olive oil and 1 tablespoon balsamic vinegar

DINNER (SLOW FUEL)

Vegan Slow Cooker Chili (page 145)

SNACK 1 (SLOW FUEL)

Handful of almonds
Assorted chopped raw vegetables

SNACK 2 (SLOW FUEL)

8 ounces **Fuelin' Veggie Juice 2 (page 174)**

DAY 5

BREAKFAST (SLOW FUEL)

1 cup non-dairy yogurt
Handful of almonds

LUNCH (SLOW FUEL)

Leftover **Vegan Slow Cooker Chili (page 145)**

DINNER (FAST FUEL)

Veggie Enchiladas (page 89) (use a non-dairy shredded cheese in place of the Mexican cheese)

SNACK 1 (SLOW FUEL)

Handful of pumpkin seeds
1 cup almond milk

SNACK 2 (SLOW FUEL)

Almond Delight Smoothie (page 169)

DAY 6

BREAKFAST (SLOW FUEL)

Tofu scrambled with chopped tomatoes, onions, and green bell pepper slices in 1 tablespoon olive oil

LUNCH (SLOW FUEL)

Leftover **Veggie Enchiladas (page 89)**

DINNER (FAST FUEL)

Light Meatless Spaghetti (page 88)

SNACK 1 (SLOW FUEL)

Almond Delight Smoothie (page 169)

SNACK 2 (SLOW FUEL)

Handful of almonds
Assorted raw cut-up slow-fuel vegetables

DAY 7

BREAKFAST (SLOW FUEL)

2 veggie sausage patties, pan-fried
1 tomato, sliced

LUNCH (FAST FUEL)

Leftover **Light Meatless Spaghetti (page 88)**

DINNER (SLOW FUEL)

Veggie burger, pan-fried
1 cup stewed tomatoes

SNACK 1 (SLOW FUEL)

2 ounces non-dairy cheese
1 cup kale chips

SNACK 2 (SLOW FUEL)

Almond Delight Smoothie (page 169)

SHOPPING LIST FOR SAMPLE PLANT-BASED BLOCK 1: MAIN INGREDIENTS

VEGETABLES

1 package frozen stir-fry vegetables

1 package alfalfa sprouts

1 bunch celery

2 red onions

2–3 yellow onions

Two 16-ounce bags fresh spinach

One 16-ounce bag fresh kale

Two 16-ounce bags mixed greens (for salads)

1 bag baby carrots

4–5 cucumbers

1 package carrots

1–2 red bell peppers

3–4 green bell peppers

1 package fresh dill

1 package fresh mint

1 package fresh basil

1 bunch cilantro

2 tomatoes

Two 15-ounce cans diced tomatoes and green chiles

One 28-ounce can crushed tomatoes

1 package broccoli and cauliflower florets

3–4 portobello mushroom caps

One 15-ounce can corn

1 bunch parsley

1 bunch asparagus

One 15-ounce can garbanzo beans

One 15-ounce can black beans

One 15-ounce can plum tomatoes

One 15-ounce can stewed tomatoes

1 bottle tomato juice

FRUITS

1 small carton fresh blueberries

3 bananas

2 small cans pineapple chunks in juice

NON-DAIRY AND MEAT SUBSTITUTES

1–2 cartons unsweetened almond milk

1 package faux chicken strips

1 carton firm tofu

1 large package imitation ground meat (textured vegetable protein)

1 package veggie burgers

One 8-ounce carton non-dairy yogurt

1 package veggie sausage patties

BREADS, CEREALS, PASTA, AND GRAINS

1 box whole-wheat pasta

1 package whole-wheat tortillas

MISCELLANEOUS

1 package chili seasoning

Two 8-ounce packages unsweetened
   frozen açai puree

Two 15-ounce cans enchilada sauce

1 small bottle white wine

1 jar almond butter

1 carton coconut water

ACKNOWLEDGMENTS

Publishing 125 easy-to-prepare, tasty, and unique recipes that neatly fit into the Body Fuel plan was a daunting project given my exceptional plainness of taste that has always allowed me to sustain a healthful diet with very little variety. With the help of military dining facilities that reliably serves four hot meals per day, my trainees were also easily able to follow my nutritional guidance without much need for culinary creativity. Had it not been for the tireless, innovative, and tasteful work of Samantha Nomany, *You Are Your Own Gym: The Cookbook* would have been a very different product. For over six months, she burned the candle at both ends to create, test, tweak, and again test the many recipes in this book, while also handling the operational management of my company. It's because of Samantha's immense contribution, with the support of her assistant Anne Nguyen, that the recipes in this book and the 3-Block System in Body Fuel can now be enjoyed with little effort by the very broad and culturally varied audience of *You Are Your Own Gym.*

REFERENCES

Bazzano, L. A., et al. 2014. Effects of low-carbohydrate and low-fat diets: a randomized trial. *Annals of Internal Medicine* 161:309–318.

Davoodi, S. H., et al. 2014. Calorie shifting diet versus calorie restriction diet: a comparative clinical trial study. *International Journal of Preventive Medicine* 5:447–456.

Kratz, M., et al. 2013. The relationship between high-fat dairy consumption and obesity, cardiovascular, and metabolic disease. *European Journal of Nutrition* 52:1–24.

McAfee, A. J., et al. 2011. Red meat from animals offered a grass diet increases plasma and platelet n-3 PUFA in healthy consumers. *British Journal of Nutrition* 105:80–89.

Ostman, E. M., et al. 2001. Inconsistency between glycemic and insulinemic responses to regular and fermented milk products. *American Journal of Clinical Nutrition* 74:96–100.

Roosevelt, M. 2006. The grass-fed revolution. Beef raised wholly on pasture, rather than grain-fed in feedlots, may be better for your health—and for the planet. *Time*, June 12, 76–78.

Siri-Tarino, P. W., et al. 2010. Saturated fat, carbohydrate, and cardiovascular disease. *American Journal of Clinical Nutrition* 91:502–509.

Wolfson, J. A., and S. N. Bleich. 2015. Is cooking at home associated with better diet quality or weight-loss intention? *Public Health Nutrition* 18:1397–1406.

Vander Wal, J. S., et al. 2005. Short-term effect of eggs on satiety in overweight and obese subjects. *Journal of the American College of Nutrition* 24:510–515.

INDEX

Page numbers in **boldface** refer to recipes.

A

açai berries:
Tropical Açai Bowl, **33,** 208, 237, 244, 249–50
Acorn Squash with Turkey Sausage, **69**
almond butter:
Almond Butter and Jelly Rice Cakes, **96,** 206, 238
No-Bake Almond Butter Banana Bites, **190,** 214, 224
No-Bake Almond Butter Squares, **183**
Almond Butter and Jelly Rice Cakes, **96**
menu plans and, 206, 238
Almond Delight Smoothie, **169**
block 1 menu plans and, 230–33
block 2 menu plans and, 219, 225
block 3 menu plans and, 208, 214
plant-based diet and, 238, 243–45, 249–52
as slow-fuel beverage, 155
almond milk:
Almond Delight Smoothie, **169,** 208, 214, 219, 225, 238, 243–45, 249–52
as non-dairy food, 19, 154
Pumpkin Protein Smoothie, **160,** 206
Strawberry and Pineapple Smoothie, **162,** 207, 238, 249
almonds:
Blended Super Juice, **172,** 208, 243
as source of protein, 18
Strawberry and Pineapple Smoothie, **162,** 207, 238, 249

American Dietetic Association, 26
Annals of Internal Medicine, 7–8
antioxidants, 16–18, 33
Apple Melontini Smoothie, **166**
apples:
Apple Melontini Smoothie, **166**
Blended Super Juice, **172,** 208, 243
Chicken Coleslaw Salad, **37,** 208
the Hulk Smoothie, **165,** 200, 225
No-Bake Chocolate Apple Oatmeal Cookies, **182,** 209
Asian cuisine:
Asian Ginger Chicken, **126**
Five-Spice Pork Chops, **87,** 202, 206
Mushrooms, Tofu, and Baby Bok Choy, **142,** 240, 245
Pad Thai with Kelp Noodles, **121**
Thai Green Chicken Curry, **74**
Tofu Orzo Bowl, **57,** 237, 245
veggies and, 83
Asian Ginger Chicken, **126,** 218
asparagus, 36, 102
Athletic Omelet, **105**
menu plans and, 221, 225, 232
avocado:
Blended Super Juice, **172,** 208, 243
Crabmeat-Stuffed Avocado, **149,** 212
Tex-Mex Corn and Avocado Salad, **50,** 202

B

baby bok choy, 142
bacon:
Bacon Scrambled over Asparagus, **102,** 220
Baked Potatoes with Eggs, **29,** 212, 215, 226
Corn Chowder with Shrimp and Bacon, **111,** 230

Tex-Mex Corn and Avocado Salad, **50,** 202
Bacon Scrambled over Asparagus, **102,** 220
Baked Broccoli and Cheddar Frittata, **103,** 231
Baked Egg in a Hole, **25**
meal plans and, 200, 206, 213, 230
Baked Potatoes with Eggs, **29**
meal plans and, 212, 215, 226
Baked Salmon Fish Sticks, **95**
Balsamic Chicken, **136**
Banana Blueberry Cookies, **184**
meal plans and, 208
plant-based diet and, 239–40
bananas:
Banana Blueberry Cookies, **184,** 208, 239–40
Chocolate Banana Protein Cupcakes, **191,** 201
how to freeze, 157
No-Bake Almond Butter Banana Bites, **190,** 214, 224
smoothies and, 156–61, 173
Sunshine Sorbet, **194,** 219, 231, 239–40
barbecue sauce, 21, 42
basil:
Ham Pesto Zoodles, **141,** 218, 225
Herbed Chicken Breasts, **137,** 230
Watermelon Basil, **179**
see also pesto
beans:
Chicken and White Bean Soup, **46,** 221, 238
green beans and, 137
as source of protein, 6
Tex-Mex Corn and Avocado Salad, **50,** 202
Vegan Lentil Salad, **107,** 239, 244, 249–51
Veggie Enchiladas, **89,** 238, 244, 251

beef:
    Easy Linguine with Meat Sauce, **84,** 233
    Filet Mignon Skewers, **144**
    Ginger Beef, **83,** 200, 208, 213
    Pesto Steak Sandwich, **54,** 212
    as source of protein, 6
    Tri-Tip and Broccolini, **138,** 219
beets:
    Just Beet It Juice, **175,** 207
berries, *see* fruits and berries
beverages, slow-fuel:
    Almond Delight Smoothie, **169,** 208, 214, 219, 225, 238, 243–45, 249–52
    Fuelin' Veggie Juice 2, 155, **174,** 200, 206, 212, 218, 221, 226, 230, 237, 243, 246, 249–50
    vs. fast-fuel, 155
black beans, 50, 89
Blackened Grouper and Snap Peas, **130,** 219
blended juices, 172–74
Blended Super Juice, **172**
    meal plans and, 208, 243
block 1 meal plans:
    daily, 198
    plant-based, 249–52
    sample, 10
    weekly, 230–33
block 2 meal plans:
    daily, 197
    plant-based, 243–46
    sample, 10
    week 1, 218–21
    week 2, 224–27
block 3 meal plans:
    daily, 196
    plant-based, 237–40
    sample, 9
    week 1, 200–203
    week 2, 206–9
    week 3, 212–15
blueberries:
    Banana Blueberry Cookies, **184,** 208, 239–40
    Blueberry Dream Smoothie, **157,** 202, 237, 245
    Complete Morning Glory, **26,** 201, 213
    Sunrise Smoothie, **156,** 207, 218, 226, 231

Blueberry Dream Smoothie, **157**
    meal plans and, 202, 237, 245
Body by You (Lauren), 7
body fuel, 14
Body Fuel (Lauren), 4, 7, 195
breads:
    English muffins, 30–32
    as fast-fuel carb, 9, 17
    rye, 55
    tortillas, 42, 47, 89
    whole-grain, 35, 41
    whole-wheat, 25–26, 31
Breakfast Cups:
    meal plans and, 224, 232
    recipe for, **99**
breakfasts, fast-fuel:
    Baked Egg in a Hole, **25,** 200, 206, 213, 230
    Baked Potatoes with Eggs, **29,** 212, 215, 226
    Broccoli and Goat Cheese Omelet with Toast, **31,** 202, 212, 219
    Complete Morning Glory, **26,** 201, 213
    Hangover Breakfast Sandwich, **32,** 202
    meal plans and, 166
    Sunrise Egg Muffin, **30,** 201, 208, 227
    Tropical Açaí Bowl, **33,** 208, 237, 244, 249–50
breakfasts, slow-fuel:
    Athletic Omelet, **105,** 221, 225, 232
    Bacon Scrambled over Asparagus, **102,** 210
    Baked Broccoli and Cheddar Frittata, **103,** 231
    Breakfast Cups, **99**
    Egg and Squash Skillet, **100,** 219
    Eggs in a Nest, **101,** 220, 233
    Smoked Gouda and Veggie Frittata, **104**
    Smoked Ham and Spinach Quiche, **106**
broccoli:
    Baked Broccoli and Cheddar Frittata, **103,** 231
    Broccoli and Goat Cheese Omelet with Toast, **31,** 202, 212, 219

    Green Goddess Smoothie, **173,** 201, 250
Broccoli and Goat Cheese Omelet with Toast, **31**
    meal plans and, 202, 212, 219
broccolini:
    Garlic Chicken Broccolini Salad, **119,** 232
    Tri-Tip and Broccolini, **138,** 219
broth, 21, 45–46, 111
Brown Derby restaurant, 115
brown rice, 62, 70, 83, 85
bulk cooking, 99
butter and oils, 19–20
    see also almond butter

C

cabbage:
    Chicken Coleslaw Salad, **37,** 208
    Vietnamese Chicken Salad, **118,** 225
calorie cycling, 4, 8–11
cannellini beans, 46
capers, 21, 66
carbohydrates, fast-fuel, *see* fast-fuel carbs
carbohydrates, slow-fuel, *see* slow-fuel carbs
carrots:
    Apple Melontini Smoothie, **166**
    Protein Carrot Cake Bites, **188**
Cauliflower Casserole, **148,** 231
Cauliflower Skillet, **139**
cereals, 17
    see also oats
cheddar cheese:
    Athletic Omelet, **105,** 221, 225, 232
    Baked Broccoli and Cheddar Frittata, **103,** 231
    Cauliflower Casserole, **148,** 231
    Cheeseburger Macaroni, **81**
cheese:
    Athletic Omelet, **105,** 221, 225, 232
    Baked Broccoli and Cheddar Frittata, **103,** 231

Broccoli and Goat Cheese Omelet with Toast, **31,** 202, 212, 219

Cauliflower Casserole, **148,** 231

Cheeseburger Macaroni, **81**

Chicken Parmesan with Spaghetti Squash, **134,** 231–32

Low-Fat Lasagna, **79,** 220

Pesto Chicken Bake, **135**

Smoked Gouda and Veggie Frittata, **104**

Spaghetti Squash with Mediterranean Scramble, **147**

Cheeseburger Macaroni, **81**

chia seeds:

Chocolate Strawberry Chia Pudding, **187,** 213–14

Strawberry Smoothie, **158,** 202

uses for, 160

chicken:

Asian Ginger Chicken, **126**

Balsamic Chicken, **136**

Chicken and Spinach Pizza, **75**

Chicken and Veggie Pasta, **76**

Chicken and White Bean Soup, **46,** 221, 238

Chicken Capers with Orzo, **66**

Chicken Coleslaw Salad, **37,** 208

Chicken Curry Wraps, **41,** 206

Chicken Kale Soup, **45,** 203, 218

Chicken Orzo Salad, **38,** 200, 214

Chicken Parmesan with Spaghetti Squash, **134,** 231–32

Chicken Schnitzel, **67,** 207

Chicken with Strawberries and Spinach Salad, **51,** 206

Chicken Zoodles Chow Mein, **128,** 230

Garlic Chicken Broccolini Salad, **119,** 232

Hawaiian BBQ Chicken Pizza, **42,** 219

Herbed Chicken Breasts, **137,** 230

Mediterranean Chicken Kabobs, **73**

Mediterranean Chicken Wraps, **47,** 202

Pad Thai with Kelp Noodles, **121**

Pesto Chicken Bake, **135**

Slow Cooker Chicken and Rice, **70**

Tandoori Chicken and Cucumber Salad, **131**

Thai Green Chicken Curry, **74**

Vietnamese Chicken Salad, **118,** 225

Chicken and Spinach Pizza, **75**

Chicken and Veggie Pasta, **76**

Chicken and White Bean Soup, **46**

menu plans and, 221

plant-based diet and, 238

chicken broth:

Chicken and White Bean Soup, **46,** 221, 238

Corn Chowder with Shrimp and Bacon, **111,** 230

Chicken Capers with Orzo, **66**

Chicken Coleslaw Salad, **37,** 208

Chicken Curry Wraps, **41,** 206

Chicken Kale Soup, **45**

meal plans and, 203, 218

recipe for, 45

Chicken Orzo Salad, **38**

meal plans and, 200, 214

Chicken Parmesan with Spaghetti Squash, **34**

meal plans and, 231–32

Chicken Schnitzel, **67,** 207

Chicken with Strawberries and Spinach Salad, **51,** 206

Chicken Zoodles Chow Mein, **128,** 230

chiles, 90

Chinese cuisine, 20

chocolate:

Almond Delight Smoothie, **169,** 208, 214, 219, 225, 238, 243–45, 249–52

Chocolate Banana Protein Cupcakes, **191,** 201

Chocolate Strawberry Chia Pudding, **187,** 213–14

No-Bake Chocolate Apple Oatmeal Cookies, **182,** 209

Chocolate Banana Protein Cupcakes, **191,** 201

Chocolate Strawberry Chia Pudding, **187,** 213–14

Cholula Hot Sauce, 21, 89

cilantro, 60

Cobb, Robert Howard, 115

coconut, 188

coconut milk:

Chocolate Strawberry Chia Pudding, **187,** 213–14

as non-dairy food, 19, 154

coconut water, 173

collard greens, 172

comfort foods, 81, 191

Complete Morning Glory, **26**

meal plans and, 201, 213

condiments, 21, 94, 136

see also sauces

Consumer Reports, 85

cooking methods, 130–31

Coriander Baked Salmon, **60**

meal plans and, 200, 209

corn:

Corn Chowder with Shrimp and Bacon, **111,** 230

Tex-Mex Corn and Avocado Salad, **50,** 202

Corn Chowder with Shrimp and Bacon, **111,** 230

Crabmeat-Stuffed Avocado, **149,** 212

Cream of Wheat Soup, **55**

Cuban cuisine, 78

cucumbers:

blended juices and, 172–73

Cucumber Tuna Boats, **151,** 207–8, 219, 231

Mediterranean Chicken Wraps, **47,** 202

Refreshing Cucumber Salad with Tuna, **108,** 230

Tandoori Chicken and Cucumber Salad, **131**

uses for, 109

Cucumber Tuna Boats, **151**

meal plans and, 207–8, 219, 231

cumin, 20, 89

curry:

Chicken Curry Wraps, **41,** 206

Slow Cooker Indian Lamb Curry, **85,** 201, 208–9

Thai Green Chicken Curry, **74**

D

dairy foods, *see* cheese; yogurt

dates, 184

desserts, fast-fuel:
  Banana Blueberry Cookies, **184,** 208, 239–40
  Chocolate Banana Protein Cupcakes, **191,** 201
  Chocolate Strawberry Chia Pudding, **187,** 213–14
  No-Bake Almond Butter Banana Bites, **190,** 214, 224
  No-Bake Almond Butter Squares, **183**
  No-Bake Chocolate Apple Oatmeal Cookies, **182,** 209
  Protein Carrot Cake Bites, **188**
  Strawberry Frozen Yogurt, **193,** 214–15, 226–27
  Sunshine Sorbet, **194,** 219, 231, 239–40
dietary fat, 8
diet plateauing, 4, 9
dill, 20, 132
dinners, fast-fuel:
  Acorn Squash with Turkey Sausage, **69**
  Cheeseburger Macaroni, **81**
  Chicken and Veggie Pasta, **76**
  Chicken Capers with Orzo, **66**
  Chicken Schnitzel, **67,** 207
  Coriander Baked Salmon, **60,** 200, 209
  Easy Linguine with Meat Sauce, **84,** 233
  Edamame Spaghetti and Shrimp, **63**
  Five-Spice Pork Chops, **87,** 202, 206
  Ginger Beef, **83,** 200, 208, 213
  Ginger Sea Bass, **59,** 203, 206
  Gnocchi and Smoked Turkey Sausage, **77**
  Light Meatless Spaghetti, **88,** 239, 243–46, 252
  Low-Fat Lasagna, **79,** 220
  Mediterranean Chicken Kabobs, **73**
  Quinoa and Turkey Chorizo–Stuffed Chiles, **90,** 220–21
  Salmon Pasta, 65
  Sesame Seared Ahi Tuna, **62**
  Slow Cooker Chicken and Rice, **70**

  Slow Cooker Indian Lamb Curry, **85,** 201, 208–9
  Spicy Shrimp and Wild Rice, **61,** 201
  Thai Green Chicken Curry, **74**
  Turkey Picadillo, **78,** 212
  Veggie Enchiladas, **89,** 238, 244, 251
dinners, slow-fuel:
  Asian Ginger Chicken, **126**
  Balsamic Chicken, **136**
  Blackened Grouper and Snap Peas, **130,** 219
  Cauliflower Casserole, **148,** 231
  Cauliflower Skillet, **139**
  Chicken Parmesan with Spaghetti Squash, **134,** 231–32
  Chicken Zoodles Chow Mein, **128,** 230
  Filet Mignon Skewers, **144**
  Grilled Rosemary Lamb Chops, **125**
  Ham Pesto Zoodles, **141,** 218, 225
  Herbed Chicken Breasts, **137,** 230
  Mushrooms, Tofu, and Baby Bok Choy, **142,** 240, 245
  Pesto Chicken Bake, **135**
  Spaghetti Squash with Mediterranean Scramble, **147**
  Tandoori Chicken and Cucumber Salad, **131**
  Tilapia and Dill in Parchment, **132**
  Tri-Tip and Broccolini, **138,** 219
  Vegan Slow Cooker Chili, **145,** 243–46, 250

E

Easy Linguine with Meat Sauce, **84,** 233
Edamame Spaghetti and Shrimp, **63**
Egg and Squash Skillet, **100,** 219
eggs:
  Egg and Squash Skillet, **100,** 219
  Eggs in a Nest, **101,** 220, 233
  fast-fuel breakfasts and, 25–32

  frittatas and, 103–4
  omelets and, 31, 105
  quiche and, 106
  skillets and, 100, 139, 219
  slow-fuel breakfasts and, 99–106
  as snacks, 150
  as source of protein, 6, 15, 191
  as staple, 15
Eggs in a Nest, **101**
  meal plans and, 220, 233
egg whites, 29, 95
elbow macaroni, 81
English muffins:
  Hangover Breakfast Sandwich, **32,** 202
  Sunrise Egg Muffin, **30,** 201, 208, 227
European Journal of Nutrition, 19
exercise, 4–7
  see also post-workout refueling

F

farfalle (bow-tie pasta), 65
fast-fuel breakfasts:
  Baked Egg in a Hole, **25,** 200, 206, 213, 230
  Baked Potatoes with Eggs, **29,** 212, 215, 226
  Broccoli and Goat Cheese Omelet with Toast, **31,** 202, 212, 219
  Complete Morning Glory, **26,** 201, 213
  Hangover Breakfast Sandwich, **32,** 202
  meal plans and, 166
  Sunrise Egg Muffin, **30,** 201, 208, 227
  Tropical Açai Bowl, **33,** 208, 237, 244, 249–50
fast-fuel carbs:
  bread as, 9, 17
  exercise and, 6
  pasta as, 9, 17
  potatoes as, 9
  rice as, 9, 62, 83–85
  vs. slow-fuel, 4–6
  weight loss and, 10

fast-fuel desserts:
    Banana Blueberry Cookies, **184,** 208, 239–40
    Chocolate Banana Protein Cupcakes, **191,** 201
    Chocolate Strawberry Chia Pudding, **187,** 213–14
    No-Bake Almond Butter Banana Bites, **190,** 214, 224
    No-Bake Almond Butter Squares, **183**
    No-Bake Chocolate Apple Oatmeal Cookies, **182,** 209
    Protein Carrot Cake Bites, **188**
    Strawberry Frozen Yogurt, **193,** 214–15, 226–27
    Sunshine Sorbet, **194,** 219, 231, 239–40
fast fuel dinners:
    Acorn Squash with Turkey Sausage, **69**
    Cheeseburger Macaroni, **81**
    Chicken and Veggie Pasta, **76**
    Chicken Capers with Orzo, **66**
    Chicken Schnitzel, **67,** 207
    Coriander Baked Salmon, **60,** 200, 209
    Easy Linguine with Meat Sauce, **84,** 233
    Edamame Spaghetti and Shrimp, **63**
    Five-Spice Pork Chops, **87,** 202, 206
    Ginger Beef, **83,** 200, 208, 213
    Ginger Sea Bass, **59,** 203, 206
    Gnocchi and Smoked Turkey Sausage, **77**
    Light Meatless Spaghetti, **88,** 239, 243–46, 252
    Low-Fat Lasagna, **79,** 220
    Mediterranean Chicken Kabobs, **73**
    Quinoa and Turkey Chorizo-Stuffed Chiles, **90,** 220–21
    Salmon Pasta, 65
    Sesame Seared Ahi Tuna, **62**
    Slow Cooker Chicken and Rice, **70**
    Slow Cooker Indian Lamb Curry, **85,** 201, 208–9
    Spicy Shrimp and Wild Rice, **61,** 201

    Thai Green Chicken Curry, **74**
    Turkey Picadillo, **78,** 212
    Veggie Enchiladas, **89,** 238, 244, 251
fast-fuel lunches:
    Chicken and White Bean Soup, **46,** 221, 238
    Chicken Coleslaw Salad, **37,** 208
    Chicken Curry Wraps, **41,** 206
    Chicken Kale Soup, **45,** 203, 218
    Chicken Orzo Salad, **38,** 200, 214
    Chicken with Strawberries and Spinach Salad, **51,** 206
    Cream of Wheat Soup, **55**
    Guilt-Free Sloppy Joe, **49,** 201, 207
    Hawaiian BBQ Chicken Pizza, **42,** 219
    Mediterranean Chicken Wraps, **47,** 202
    Pesto Steak Sandwich, **54,** 212
    Salmon Salad Sandwich, **35,** 200, 213, 220
    Salmon Soba Noodle Bowl, **36,** 218
    Southwestern Orzo Salad, **52,** 219
    Tex-Mex Corn and Avocado Salad, **50,** 202
    Tofu Orzo Bowl, **57,** 237, 245
fast-fuel meals:
    breakfasts and, 24–33
    dinners and, 58–91
    lunches and, 34–57
fast-fuel snacks, 92–96
fast-fuel veggies, 16
fat burning, 4–7, 10, 16, 19
fat fuel, 7–8
feta cheese, 147
fiber, 5, 18, 50, 69, 91
figs, 51
Filet Mignon Skewers, **144,** 226
fish:
    Baked Salmon Fish Sticks, **95**
    Blackened Grouper and Snap Peas, **130,** 219
    Coriander Baked Salmon, **60,** 200, 209
    Cucumber Tuna Boats, **151,** 207–8, 219, 231
    Ginger Sea Bass, **59,** 203, 206

    Refreshing Cucumber Salad with Tuna, **108,** 230
    Salmon Pasta, 65
    Salmon Salad Sandwich, **35,** 200, 213, 220
    Salmon Soba Noodle Bowl, **36,** 218
    Sesame Seared Ahi Tuna, **62**
    as source of protein, 6, 15
    as staple, 15, 35
    Stuffed Eggs, **150,** 202, 213, 224–25, 230–31
    Tilapia and Dill in Parchment, **132**
    Zucchini and Salmon Salad, **112,** 231
Five-Spice Pork Chops, **87**
    meal plans and, 202, 206
food budget, 11
free-range poultry, 14–15
frittatas, 103–4
fruits and berries:
    açai berries, 33
    apples, 37, 165, 166, 172, 182
    bananas, 156–61, 173, 184, 190–91, 194
    blueberries, 26, 156–57, 184
    calorie cycling and, 16–17
    dates, 184
    figs, 51
    grapefruit, 176
    mango, 167, 194
    oranges, 156
    peaches, 163
    pears, 165
    pineapple, 159, 162, 172
    raspberries, 178
    strawberries, 26, 51, 96, 158, 162, 187, 193
    tangerines, 50
    watermelon, 179
fuel blocks:
    block 1 day, 198
    block 1 sample, 10
    block 1 week 1, 230–33
    block 2 day, 197
    block 2 sample, 10
    block 2 week 1, 218–21
    block 2 week 2, 224–27
    block 3 day, 196
    block 3 sample, 9
    block 3 week 1, 200–203

fuel blocks (*cont.*):
    block 3 week 2, 206–9
    block 3 week 3, 212–15
    calorie cycling and, 8–11
    plant-based block 1, 249–52
    plant-based block 2, 243–46
    plant-based block 3, 237–40
    see also meal planning
Fuelin' Veggie Juice 2, **174**
    block 1 meal plans and, 230
    block 2 meal plans and, 218, 221, 226
    block 3 meal plans and, 200, 206, 212
    plant-based diet and, 237, 243, 246, 249–50
    as slow-fuel beverage, 155

G
garam masala, 20, 85
garlic:
    Garlic Chicken Broccolini Salad, **119**, 232
    Ginger Beef, **83,** 200, 208, 213
    Herbed Chicken Breasts, **137,** 230
    see also Italian cuisine
Garlic Chicken Broccolini Salad, **119**, 232
genetically modified ingredients (GMOs), 16
German cuisine:
    Chicken Schnitzel, **67**, 207
    Cream of Wheat Soup, **55**
ginger:
    Asian Ginger Chicken, **126**
    Ginger Beef, **83,** 200, 208, 213
    Ginger Sea Bass, **59**, 203, 206
    Green with Envy Juice, **170,** 239
    Mango Ginger Smoothie, **167,** 214, 232
Ginger Beef, **83**
    meal plans and, 200, 208, 213
Ginger Sea Bass, **59**
    meal plans and, 203, 206
gluten-free foods, 17, 63, 91, 188
glycemic index, 5
glycemic load, 5

Gnocchi and Smoked Turkey Sausage, **77**
goat cheese, 31
Gouda cheese, 104
grains, 17, 35, 41
    see also quinoa; rice
grapefruit, 176
grass-fed meats, 14–15, 54
Greek cuisine, 147
green drinks, 170–73
Green Goddess Smoothie, **173**
    meal plans and, 201, 250
greens, leafy, 164–65
    see also kale; lettuce; spinach
Green with Envy Juice, **170,** 239
Green Zen Smoothie, **164**
    meal plans and, 203, 212, 237, 244
Grilled Rosemary Lamb Chops, **125**
Grilled Shrimp and Spinach Salad, **114,** 220
Guilt-Free Sloppy Joe, **49**
    menu plans and, 201, 207

H
Ham Pesto Zoodles, **141**
    meal plans and, 218, 225
Hangover Breakfast Sandwich, **32,** 202
Hawaiian BBQ Chicken Pizza, **42,** 219
Herbed Chicken Breasts, **137,** 230
herbs and spices, 20, 61, 137
    see also individual herbs and spices
Hulk Smoothie, the, **165**
    meal plans and, 200, 225

I
Indian cuisine:
    Slow Cooker Indian Lamb Curry, **85,** 201, 208–9
    Tandoori Chicken and Cucumber Salad, **131**
    turmeric and, 20

Italian cuisine:
    Chicken Parmesan with Spaghetti Squash, **134,** 231–32
    Easy Linguine with Meat Sauce, **84,** 233
    Gnocchi and Smoked Turkey Sausage, **77**
    Ham Pesto Zoodles, **141,** 218, 225
    Herbed Chicken Breasts, **137,** 230
    Low-Fat Lasagna, **79**, 220
    Pesto Steak Sandwich, **54,** 212

J
Japanese cuisine:
    miso and, 126–27
    Salmon Soba Noodle Bowl, **36,** 218
    Sesame Seared Ahi Tuna, **62**
jasmine rice, 74
juices:
    blended juices and, 172–74
    Fuelin' Veggie Juice 2, 155, **174,** 200, 206, 212, 218, 221, 226, 230, 237, 243, 246, 249–50
    Just Beet It Juice, **175,** 207
    Raspberry Tang Juice, **178,** 209
    Red Grapefruit Juice, **176,** 207
    Super Juice, **172**
    Watermelon Basil Juice, **179,** 214
    see also smoothies
Just Beet It Juice, **175,** 207

K
kabobs, 73
kale:
    Chicken Kale Soup, **45,** 203, 218
    Green Goddess Smoothie, **173,** 201, 250
    Green with Envy Juice, **170,** 239
    as super green, 45, 164
kelp noodles, 121
kitchen equipment, 21–22, 128–29

L

lacto-ovo-vegetarian, 236
lactose-free foods, 19, 31, 154, 188
lacto-vegetarian, 236
lamb:
Grilled Rosemary Lamb Chops, **125**
Slow Cooker Indian Lamb Curry, **85,** 201, 208–9
as source of protein, 6
lasagna, 79
Latin American cuisine, 78
lentils, 107
lettuce:
Spicy Shrimp and Cobb Salad, **115,** 227
as super green, 164
Taco Lettuce Boats, **123,** 224
Turkey Lettuce Wraps, **122,** 231, 233
leucine, 7
Light Meatless Spaghetti, **88**
meal plans and, 239, 243–46, 252
linguine, 84
Low-Fat Lasagna, **79,** 220
lunches, fast-fuel:
Chicken and White Bean Soup, **46,** 221, 238
Chicken Coleslaw Salad, **37,** 208
Chicken Curry Wraps, **41,** 206
Chicken Kale Soup, **45,** 203, 218
Chicken Orzo Salad, **38,** 200, 214
Chicken with Strawberries and Spinach Salad, **51,** 206
Cream of Wheat Soup, **55**
Guilt-Free Sloppy Joe, **49,** 201, 207
Hawaiian BBQ Chicken Pizza, **42,** 219
Mediterranean Chicken Wraps, **47,** 202
Pesto Steak Sandwich, **54,** 212
Salmon Salad Sandwich, **35,** 200, 213, 220
Salmon Soba Noodle Bowl, **36,** 218
Southwestern Orzo Salad, **52,** 219

Tex-Mex Corn and Avocado Salad, **50,** 202
Tofu Orzo Bowl, **57,** 237, 245
lunches, slow-fuel:
Corn Chowder with Shrimp and Bacon, **111,** 230
Garlic Chicken Broccolini Salad, **119,** 232
Grilled Shrimp and Spinach Salad, **114,** 220
Pad Thai with Kelp Noodles, **121**
Refreshing Cucumber Salad with Tuna, **108,** 230
Shrimp Salad Wraps, **117,** 224
Spicy Shrimp and Cobb Salad, **115,** 227
Taco Lettuce Boats, **123,** 224
Turkey Lettuce Wraps, **122,** 231, 233
Vietnamese Chicken Salad, **118,** 225
Zucchini and Salmon Salad, **112,** 231

M

macaroni and cheese, 81
mango:
Mango Ginger Smoothie, **167,** 214, 232
Sunshine Sorbet, **194,** 219, 231, 239–40
Mango Ginger Smoothie, **167**
meal plans and, 214, 232
marinades, 125
Mark's Easy Homemade Ketchup, **94**
mayo-lemon sauce, 32
meal designs, 9–10, 199, 217, 229
meal planning:
block 1 day, 198
block 1 sample, 10
block 1 week, 230–33
block 2 day, 197
block 2 sample, 10
block 2 week 1, 218–21
block 2 week 2, 224–27
block 3 day, 196
block 3 sample, 9

block 3 week 1, 200–203
block 3 week 2, 206–9
block 3 week 3, 212–15
plant-based block 1, 249–52
plant-based block 2, 243–46
plant-based block 3, 237–40
staples and, 14–21
see also shopping lists
meal preparation, 14
meats, grass-fed, 14–15, 54
meat slicing, 83
Mediterranean Chicken Kabobs, **73**
Mediterranean Chicken Wraps, **47,** 202
Mediterranean cuisine:
Mediterranean Chicken Kabobs, **73**
Mediterranean Chicken Wraps, **47,** 202
Spaghetti Squash with Mediterranean Scramble, **147**
menus, daily, 196–98
menus, weekly:
block 1 and, 230–33
block 2 and, 218–21, 224–27
block 3 and, 200–203, 206–9, 212–215
metabolism, 4, 9, 19
Mexican cuisine:
cumin and, 20
Taco Lettuce Boats, **123,** 224
Tex-Mex Corn and Avocado Salad, **50,** 202
Veggie Enchiladas, **89,** 238, 244, 251
Middle Eastern cuisine, 73
mint leaves, 174
miso, 21, 126–27
mozzarella cheese:
Chicken Parmesan with Spaghetti Squash, **134,** 231–32
Low-Fat Lasagna, **79,** 220
Pesto Chicken Bake, **135**
muscle building, 4–9, 16, 19, 160
mushrooms:
Eggs in a Nest, **101,** 220, 233
Mushrooms, Tofu, and Baby Bok Choy, **142,** 240, 245
Mushrooms, Tofu, and Baby Bok Choy, **142**
plant-based diet and, 240, 245

N

No-Bake Almond Butter Banana
    Bites, **190**
    menu plans and, 214, 224
No-Bake Almond Butter Squares,
    183
No-Bake Chocolate Apple Oatmeal
    Cookies, **182,** 209
non-dairy foods, 19, 154, 188
noodles:
    Pad Thai with Kelp Noodles,
       121
    Salmon Soba Noodle Bowl, **36,**
       218
nutritional content, 11
nuts and seeds:
    almonds, 18, 162, 172
    chia seeds, 158, 160, 187
    coconut, 188
    as source of protein, 18, 191
    staples and, 18
    walnuts, 18, 191, 194

O

oats:
    Banana Blueberry Cookies, **184,**
       208, 239–40
    No-Bake Almond Butter Banana
       Bites, **190,** 214, 224
    No-Bake Almond Butter
       Squares, **183**
omega-3 fatty acids, 15, 158
omelets:
    Athletic Omelet, **105,** 221, 225,
       232
    Broccoli and Goat Cheese Om-
       elet with Toast, **31,** 202, 212,
       219
oranges, 156
oregano, 20, 137
organic foods, 15–17
orzo:
    Chicken Capers with
       Orzo, **66**
    Chicken Orzo Salad, **38,** 200,
       214
    Southwestern Orzo Salad, **52,**
       219
    Tofu Orzo Bowl, **57,** 237, 245

P

Pad Thai with Kelp Noodles, **121**
panko (Japanese bread
    crumbs), 93
pantry and fridge purge, 14
pasilla, 90
pasta:
    Cheeseburger Macaroni, **81**
    Chicken and Veggie Pasta, **76**
    Easy Linguine with Meat Sauce,
       84, 233
    Edamame Spaghetti and
       Shrimp, **63**
    as fast-fuel carb, 9, 17
    Light Meatless Spaghetti, **88,**
       239, 243–46, 252
    Low-Fat Lasagna, **79,** 220
    Salmon Pasta, 65
    see also noodles; orzo
Peach Pie Smoothie, **163**
    menu plans and, 200, 215
pears, 165
peppers, 73, 76
pescatarians, 236
pesticides, 17
pesto:
    Ham Pesto Zoodles, **141,** 218,
       225
    Pesto Chicken Bake, **135**
    Pesto Steak Sandwich, **54,** 212
Pesto Chicken Bake, **135**
Pesto Steak Sandwich, **54,** 212
pineapple:
    Blended Super Juice, **172,** 208,
       243
    Pineapple Power Smoothie, **159,**
       212, 224
    Strawberry and Pineapple
       Smoothie, **162,** 207, 238, 249
Pineapple Power Smoothie, **159**
    menu plans and, 212, 224
pizza:
    Chicken and Spinach Pizza, **75**
    Hawaiian BBQ Chicken Pizza,
       42, 219
plant-based diet:
    meal planning and, 237–40,
       243–46, 249–52
    protein powder and, 16
    shopping lists and, 241–42, 247–
       48, 253–54
ponzu (Japanese sauce), 21, 62

pork:
    Cauliflower Skillet, **139**
    Corn Chowder with Shrimp and
       Bacon, **111,** 230
    Five-Spice Pork Chops, **87,** 202,
       206
    Ham Pesto Zoodles, **141,** 218, 225
    as source of protein, 6
post-workout refueling:
    Almond Butter and Jelly Rice
       Cakes, **96,** 206, 238
    Apple Melontini Smoothie, **166**
    fast-fuel carbs and, 6
    Protein Carrot Cake Bites, **188**
potatoes:
    Baked Potatoes with Eggs, **29,**
       212, 215, 226
    as fast-fuel carb, 9
    Five-Spice Pork Chops, **87,** 202,
       206
    Gnocchi and Smoked Turkey
       Sausage, **77**
poultry:
    free-range, 14–15
    as source of protein, 6
    as staple, 14–15
    see also chicken; turkey
Protein Carrot Cake Bites, **188,** 220
protein fuel, 6–7, 15
protein shakes, 16, 154
    see also smoothies
Pumpkin Protein Smoothie, **160,**
    206

Q

quiche, 106
quinoa, 90–91
Quinoa and Turkey Chorizo-
    Stuffed Chiles, **90,** 220–21

R

Raspberry Tang Juice, **178,** 209
real fuel, 12
Red Grapefruit Juice, **176,** 207
Refreshing Cucumber Salad with
    Tuna, **108,** 230

rice:
    as fast-fuel carb, 9, 62, 83, 85
    Slow Cooker Chicken and
        Rice, **70**
    Spicy Shrimp and Wild Rice, **61,**
        201
    Thai Green Chicken Curry, **74**
rice cakes, 96
rice milk, 154
ricotta cheese, 79
rosemary, 20, 125
rotini (corkscrew-shaped
    pasta), 76
rye bread, 55

S

salads:
    Chicken Coleslaw Salad, **37,** 208
    Chicken Orzo Salad, **38,** 200,
        214
    Chicken with Strawberries and
        Spinach Salad, **51,** 206
    Garlic Chicken Broccolini Salad,
        119, 232
    Grilled Shrimp and Spinach
        Salad, **114,** 220
    Refreshing Cucumber Salad
        with Tuna, **108,** 230
    Southwestern Orzo Salad, **52,**
        219
    Spicy Shrimp and Cobb Salad,
        115, 227
    Tex-Mex Corn and Avocado
        Salad, **50,** 202
    Vegan Lentil Salad, **107,** 239,
        244, 249–51
    Vietnamese chicken salad, **118,**
        225
    Zucchini and Salmon Salad, **112,**
        231
salmon:
    Baked Salmon Fish Sticks, **95**
    Coriander Baked Salmon, **60,**
        200, 209
    Salmon Pasta, 65
    Salmon Salad Sandwich, **35,**
        200, 213, 220
    Salmon Soba Noodle Bowl, **36,**
        218

    Zucchini and Salmon Salad, **112,**
        231
Salmon Salad Sandwich, **35,** 200,
    213, 220
Salmon Soba Noodle Bowl, **36,** 218
salt, 20, 39
sandwiches:
    Hangover Breakfast Sandwich,
        32, 202
    liverwurst and, 55
    Pesto Steak Sandwich, **54,** 212
    Salmon Salad Sandwich, **35,**
        200, 213, 220
saturated fats, 8, 19–20, 25
sauces:
    barbecue sauce, 21, 42
    hot sauce, 21, 89
    Japanese ponzu, 21, 62
    mayo-lemon sauce, 32
    meat sauce, 84
    pesto sauce, 54, 141
    teriyaki sauce, 57
    tomato sauce, 49, 78
schnitzel:
    Chicken Schnitzel, **67,** 207
seafood:
    Corn Chowder with Shrimp and
        Bacon, **111,** 230
    Crabmeat-Stuffed Avocado,
        149, 212
    Edamame Spaghetti and
        Shrimp, **63**
    Grilled Shrimp and Spinach
        Salad, **114,** 220
    Shrimp Salad Wraps, **117,** 224
    Spicy Shrimp and Cobb Salad,
        115, 227
    Spicy Shrimp and Wild Rice, **61,**
        201
semi-vegetarian, 236
serving sizes, 198
Sesame Seared Ahi Tuna, **62**
shopping lists:
    block 1, 234–35
    block 2, 222–23, 228–29
    block 3, 204–5, 210–11, 216–17
    plant-based diet and, 241–42,
        247–48, 253–54
shrimp, *see* seafood
Shrimp Salad Wraps, **117,** 224
skillet meals:
    Cauliflower Skillet, **139**

Egg and Squash Skillet, **100,** 219
Guilt-Free Sloppy Joe, **49,** 201,
    207
sloppy joes, **49,** 201, 207
Slow Cooker Chicken and Rice, **70**
Slow Cooker Indian Lamb Curry, **85**
    meal plans and, 201, 208–9
slow cookers, 70–71, 85, 145
slow-fuel breakfasts:
    Athletic Omelet, **105,** 221, 225,
        232
    Bacon Scrambled over Aspara-
        gus, **102,** 210
    Baked Broccoli and Cheddar
        Frittata, **103,** 231
    Breakfast Cups, 99
    Egg and Squash Skillet, **100,** 219
    Eggs in a Nest, **101,** 220, 233
    Smoked Gouda and Veggie Frit-
        tata, **104**
    Smoked Ham and Spinach
        Quiche, **106**
slow-fuel carbs, 4–5
slow-fuel dinners:
    Asian Ginger Chicken, **126**
    Balsamic Chicken, **136**
    Blackened Grouper and Snap
        Peas, **130,** 219
    Cauliflower Casserole, **148,** 231
    Cauliflower Skillet, **139**
    Chicken Parmesan with Spa-
        ghetti Squash, **134,** 231–32
    Chicken Zoodles Chow Mein,
        128, 230
    Filet Mignon Skewers, **144**
    Grilled Rosemary Lamb Chops,
        125
    Ham Pesto Zoodles, **141,** 218,
        225
    Herbed Chicken Breasts, **137,**
        230
    Mushrooms, Tofu, and Baby Bok
        Choy, **142,** 240, 245
    Pesto Chicken Bake, **135**
    Spaghetti Squash with Mediter-
        ranean Scramble, **147**
    Tandoori Chicken and Cucum-
        ber Salad, **131**
    Tilapia and Dill in Parchment, **132**
    Tri-Tip and Broccolini, **138,** 219
    Vegan Slow Cooker Chili, **145,**
        243–46, 250

slow-fuel lunches:
  Corn Chowder with Shrimp and Bacon, **111,** 230
  Garlic Chicken Broccolini Salad, **119,** 232
  Grilled Shrimp and Spinach Salad, **114,** 220
  Pad Thai with Kelp Noodles, **121**
  Refreshing Cucumber Salad with Tuna, **108,** 230
  Shrimp Salad Wraps, **117,** 224
  Spicy Shrimp and Cobb Salad, **115,** 227
  Taco Lettuce Boats, **123,** 224
  Turkey Lettuce Wraps, **122,** 231, 233
  Vietnamese Chicken Salad, **118,** 225
  Zucchini and Salmon Salad, **112,** 231
slow-fuel meals:
  breakfasts, 98–106
  dinners, 124–48
  lunches, 107–23
slow-fuel snacks, 149–51
slow-fuel veggies, 16
Smoked Gouda and Veggie Frittata, 104, 225
Smoked Ham and Spinach Quiche, 106, 224
smoothies:
  Almond Delight Smoothie, **169,** 208, 214, 219, 225, 238, 243–45, 249–52
  Apple Melontini Smoothie, **166**
  Blueberry Dream Smoothie, **157,** 202, 237, 245
  Green Zen Smoothie, **164,** 203, 212, 237, 244
  the Hulk, **165,** 200, 225
  Mango Ginger Smoothie, **167,** 214, 232
  Peach Pie Smoothie, **163,** 200, 215
  Pineapple Power Smoothie, **159,** 212, 224
  Pumpkin Protein Smoothie, **160,** 206
  as source of protein, 16
  Strawberry and Pineapple Smoothie, **162,** 207, 238, 249
  Strawberry Smoothie, **158,** 202

Sunrise Smoothie, **156,** 207, 218, 226, 231
snacks, fast-fuel:
  Almond Butter and Jelly Rice Cakes, **96,** 206, 238
  Baked Salmon Fish Sticks, **95**
  Blended Super Juice, **172,** 208, 243
  Zucchini Fries, **93,** 214–15
snacks, slow-fuel:
  Crabmeat-Stuffed Avocado, **149,** 212
  Cucumber Tuna Boats, **151,** 207–8, 219, 231
  Stuffed Eggs, **150,** 202, 213, 224–25, 230–31
snap peas, 130
soba noodles, 36
sorbet, 194
soups:
  Chicken and White Bean Soup, **46,** 221, 238
  Chicken Kale Soup, **45,** 203, 218
  Corn Chowder with Shrimp and Bacon, **111,** 230
  Cream of Wheat Soup, **55**
Southeast Asian cuisine, 118
Southwestern American cuisine:
  Southwestern Orzo Salad, **52,** 219
  Tex-Mex Corn and Avocado Salad, **50,** 202
Southwestern Orzo Salad, **52,** 219
soy-based protein powders, 16
spaghetti:
  Edamame Spaghetti and Shrimp, **63**
  Light Meatless Spaghetti, **88,** 239, 243–46, 252
spaghetti squash:
  Chicken Parmesan with Spaghetti Squash, **134,** 231–32
  Spaghetti Squash with Mediterranean Scramble, **147**
Spaghetti Squash with Mediterranean Scramble, **147**
Spicy Shrimp and Cobb Salad, **115,** 227
Spicy Shrimp and Wild Rice, **61,** 201
spinach:

Blended Super Juice, **172,** 208, 243
Chicken and Spinach Pizza, **75**
Chicken with Strawberries and Spinach Salad, **51,** 206
Fuelin' Veggie Juice 2, 155, **174,** 200, 206, 212, 218, 221, 226, 230, 237, 243, 246, 249–50
Green Goddess Smoothie, **173,** 201, 250
Green Zen Smoothie, **164,** 203, 212, 237, 244
Grilled Shrimp and Spinach Salad, **114,** 220
the Hulk Smoothie, **165,** 200, 225
Just Beet It Juice, **175,** 207
Smoked Ham and Spinach Quiche, 106
as super green, 164
spiralizers, 22, 128–29
squash:
  Acorn Squash with Turkey Sausage, **69**
  Chicken Parmesan with Spaghetti Squash, **134,** 231–32
  Egg and Squash Skillet, **100,** 219
  Spaghetti Squash with Mediterranean Scramble, **147**
  yellow squash, 100, 128–29
staples:
  butter and oils, 19–20
  condiments, 21, 136
  dairy foods, 19
  eggs, 15
  fish and seafood, 15, 35
  fruits and, 16
  grain-based foods, 17
  herbs and spices, 20
  meal planning and, 14
  meat and poultry, 14–15
  nuts and seeds, 18
  protein powders, 16
  sweeteners, 18
  vegetables, 16
strawberries:
  Almond Butter and Jelly Rice Cakes, **96,** 206, 238
  Chicken with Strawberries and Spinach Salad, **51,** 206
  Chocolate Strawberry Chia Pudding, **187,** 213–14

Complete Morning Glory, **26,**
201, 213
Strawberry and Pineapple
Smoothie, **162,** 207, 238,
249
Strawberry Frozen Yogurt, **193,**
214–15, 226–27
Strawberry Smoothie, **158,** 202
Strawberry and Pineapple
Smoothie, **162**
meal plans and, 207, 238, 249
Strawberry Frozen Yogurt, **193**
meal plans and, 214–15, 226–27
Strawberry Smoothie, **158,** 202
string beans, 137
Stuffed Eggs, **150**
meal plans and, 202, 213, 224–
25, 230–31
Sunrise Egg Muffin, **30**
meal plans and, 201, 208, 227
Sunrise Smoothie, **156**
meal plans and, 207, 218, 226,
231
Sunshine Sorbet, **194**
meal plans and, 219, 231,
239–40
super greens, 45, 164
super juice, 172
sweeteners, 18, 94

T

Taco Lettuce Boats, **123,** 224
Tandoori Chicken and Cucumber
Salad, **131**
tangerines, 50
teriyaki sauce, 57
testosterone, 8
Tex-Mex Corn and Avocado Salad,
50, 202
Tex-Mex cuisine:
Southwestern Orzo Salad, **52,**
219
Tex-Mex Corn and Avocado
Salad, **50,** 202
Thai Green Chicken Curry, **74**
Tilapia and Dill in Parchment, **132**
tofu:
Mushrooms, Tofu, and Baby Bok
Choy, **142,** 240, 245

as source of protein, 6
Tofu Orzo Bowl, **57,** 237,
245
Tofu Orzo Bowl, **57**
meal plans and, 237, 245
tomatoes:
Easy Linguine with Meat Sauce,
84, 233
Gnocchi and Smoked Turkey
Sausage, **77**
Mediterranean Chicken Wraps,
47, 202
Pesto Chicken Bake, **135**
Spicy Shrimp and Cobb Salad,
115, 227
tomato juice, 174
tomato sauce, 49, 78
tortillas, 42, 47, 89
Tri-Tip and Broccolini, **138,** 219
Tropical Açai Bowl, **33**
menu plans and, 208, 237, 244,
249–50
tuna:
Cucumber Tuna Boats, **151,**
207–8, 219, 231
Refreshing Cucumber Salad
with Tuna, **108,** 230
Sesame Seared Ahi Tuna, **62**
as staple, 35
Stuffed Eggs, **150,** 202, 213,
224–25, 230–31
turkey:
Cheeseburger Macaroni, **81**
Guilt-Free Sloppy Joe, **49,** 201,
207
Taco Lettuce Boats, **123,** 224
Turkey Lettuce Wraps, **122,** 231,
233
Turkey Picadillo, **78,** 212
turkey bacon:
Baked Potatoes with Eggs, **29,**
212, 215, 226
Tex-Mex Corn and Avocado
Salad, **50,** 202
turkey chorizo, 90
turkey ham, 106
Turkey Lettuce Wraps, **122**
meal plans and, 231–33
Turkey Picadillo, **78,** 212
turkey sausage:
Acorn Squash with Turkey Sau-
sage, **69**

Complete Morning Glory, **26,**
201, 213
Gnocchi and Smoked Turkey
Sausage, **77**
turmeric, 20

U

unsaturated fats, 8, 18

V

vegan dishes:
calorie cycling and, 198
Mushrooms, Tofu, and Baby Bok
Choy, **142,** 240, 245
Vegan Lentil Salad, **107,** 239,
244, 249–51
Vegan Slow Cooker Chili, **145,**
243–46, 250
see also plant-based diet
Vegan Lentil Salad, **107**
meal plans and, 239, 244,
249–51
Vegan Slow Cooker Chili, **145**
meal plans and, 243–46,
250
vegetables:
acorn squash, 69
asparagus, 36, 102
baby bok choy, 142
beets, 175
broccoli, 31, 103, 173
broccolini, 119, 138
cabbage, 37
carrots, 166, 188
cauliflower, 139, 148
chiles, 90
collard greens, 172
corn, 50, 111
cucumbers, 47, 108–9, 131, 151,
172–73
kale, 45, 164, 170, 173
leafy greens, 164–65
lettuce, 115, 164
mushrooms, 101, 142
pumpkins, 160
snap peas, 130

vegetables (*cont.*):
spinach, 51, 75, 106, 115, 164–65, 172–75
string beans, 137
tomatoes, 47, 77, 84, 115, 135
yellow squash, 100, 128–29
zucchini, 93, 100, 112, 179
vegetarian dishes:
calorie cycling and, 198
Cauliflower Casserole, **148,** 231
Light Meatless Spaghetti, **88,** 239, 243–46, 252
Mushrooms, Tofu, and Baby Bok Choy, **142,** 240, 245
types of vegetarians and, 236
Vegan Lentil Salad, **107,** 239, 244, 249–51
Vegan Slow Cooker Chili, **145,** 243–46, 250
Veggie Enchiladas, **89,** 238, 244, 251
see also plant-based diet; smoothies
Veggie Enchiladas, **89**
meal plans and, 238, 244, 251
Vietnamese Chicken Salad, **118,** 225
Vietnamese coriander, 118
Vietnamese cuisine, 118

Sunshine Sorbet, **194,** 219, 231, 239–40
Watermelon Basil Juice, **179,** 214
weight loss, 4, 7–12
weight maintenance, 9, 12
whey-based protein powders, 16
whole foods, 12
whole-wheat bread:
Baked Egg in a Hole, **25,** 200, 206, 213, 230
Broccoli and Goat Cheese Omelet with Toast, **31,** 202, 212, 219
Complete Morning Glory, **26,** 201, 213
whole-wheat tortillas:
Hawaiian BBQ Chicken Pizza, **42,** 219
Mediterranean Chicken Wraps, **47,** 202
Veggie Enchiladas, **89,** 238, 244, 251
wild rice, 61
wraps:
Mediterranean Chicken Wraps, **47,** 202
Shrimp Salad Wraps, **117,** 224
Turkey Lettuce Wraps, **122,** 231, 233

yogurt:
Apple Melontini Smoothie, **166**
Mango Ginger Smoothie, **167,** 214, 232
Peach Pie Smoothie, **163,** 200, 215
Pineapple Power Smoothie, **159,** 212, 224
Pumpkin Protein Smoothie, **160,** 206
Strawberry Frozen Yogurt, **193,** 214–15, 226–27
Strawberry Smoothie, **158,** 202
You Are Your Own Gym (Lauren), 7, 195

Z
zoodles:
Chicken Zoodles Chow Mein, **128,** 230
Ham Pesto Zoodles, **141,** 218, 225
ways to dry, 128
zucchini:
Egg and Squash Skillet, **100,** 219
Zucchini and Salmon Salad, **112,** 231
Zucchini Fries, **93,** 214–15
see also zoodles
Zucchini and Salmon Salad, **112,** 231
Zucchini Fries, **93,** 214–15

W
walnuts:
Chocolate Banana Protein Cupcakes, **191,** 201
as source of protein, 18

Y
yellow squash:
Egg and Squash Skillet, **100,** 219
zoodles and, 128–29

ABOUT THE AUTHORS

MARK LAUREN spent fifteen years in the Special Operations community as an operator and physical training specialist. He is the author of the internationally popular body-weight bibles *You Are Your Own Gym, Body by You,* and *Body Fuel.* A sought-after personal trainer to civilian men and women of all fitness levels, he is a triathlete and former Thai boxing champion. He now lives in Phuket, Thailand.

marklauren.com
Facebook.com/bodyweight
@yourowngym

MAGGIE GREENWOOD-ROBINSON is a *New York Times* bestselling collaborator who specializes in health and fitness. She lives in Dallas, Texas.

ABOUT THE TYPE

This book was set in Gotham, a typeface designed in 2002 by Tobias Frere-Jones (b. 1970) for the Hoefler Type Foundry. Frere-Jones studied the lettering on New York City buildings to help inspire the design. Gotham is a friendly, honest, straightforward font that is neutral without being clinical, authoritative without being impersonal.